CHI KUNG
The Way of Healing

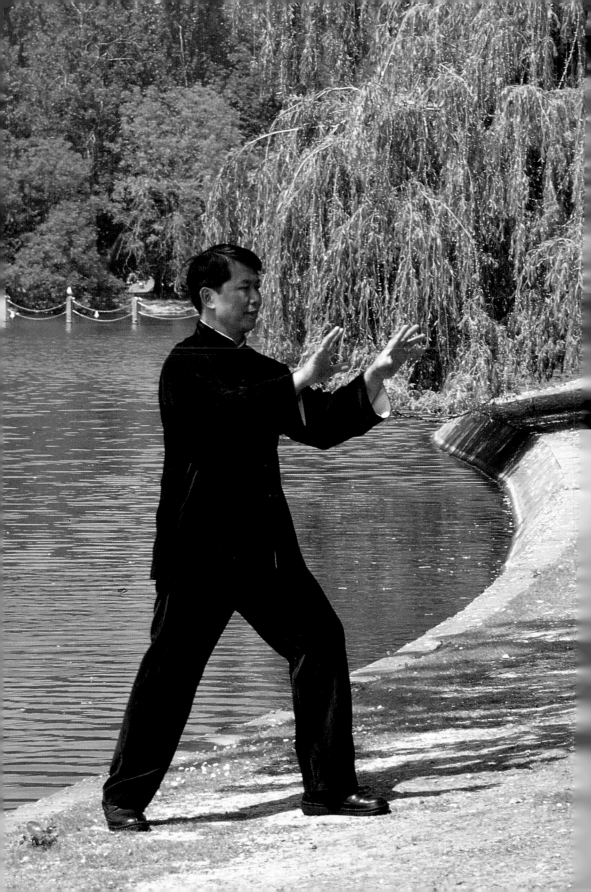

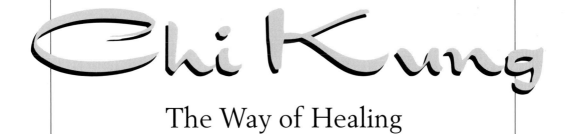

Chi Kung

The Way of Healing

 MASTER LAM KAM CHUEN

BROADWAY BOOKS   NEW YORK

BROADWAY

Broadway Books titles may be purchased for business or promotional use or for special sales. For information, please write to: Special Markets Department, Random House, Inc., 1540 Broadway, New York, NY 10036.

BROADWAY BOOKS and its logo, a letter B bisected on the diagonal, are trademarks of Broadway Books, a division of Random House, Inc.

ISBN 0-7679-0339-0

FIRST US EDITION

Designed by Bridget Morley

99 00 01 02 03 10 9 8 7 6 5 4 3 2 1

Printed and bound in Singapore.

CAUTION The techniques, ideas and suggestions in this book are not intended as a substitute for proper medical advice. Any application of the techniques, ideas and suggestions in this book is at the reader's sole discretion and risk.

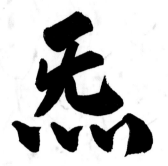

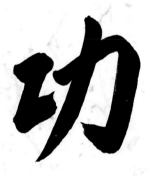

CHI KUNG

This book is dedicated
to the founder of *Zhan Zhuang* Chi Kung,
Great Grand Master Wang Xiang Zhai,
and to all those seeking health in their lives.

CONTENTS

PART FOUR

REMOVING THE OBSTACLES:
Healing yourself and Others

PART FIVE

RETURNING TO THE SOURCE:
Recovering your Health

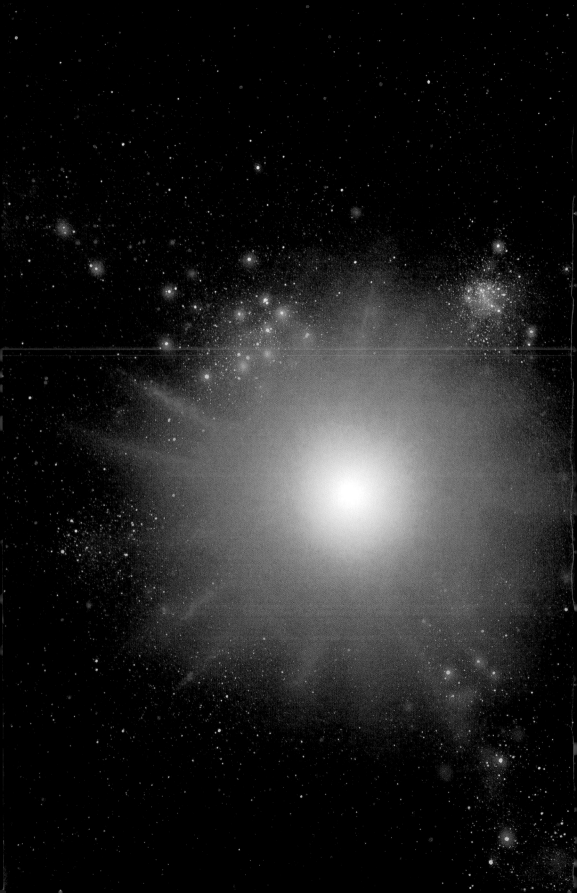

Introduction

The energy of the human body is the foundation of our health. When our energy is at its peak, our immune system is at full strength. When our energy declines we become vulnerable.

All healing depends on energy. This energy can come to us in many ways, but ultimately it is our own reserves of energy that provide the inner strength which keep us healthy and enable us to overcome illness.

Energy is the foundation of life. Without energy we die. All the cells in our bodies depend on energy for their existence. It is energy which keeps them constantly at work, reproducing and renewed.

If we learn how to increase our energy to higher levels, we can use it to support ourselves and others when we are hurt or unwell. That is what you will learn from the practices described in this book.

The energy that our bodies need is not mere fuel. Like everything else in the universe, our bodies *are* energy. We know from the most advanced scientific explorations that the universe and everything we can detect in it is a vast web of energetic forces.

This was exactly the same conclusion that the natural scientists of ancient China reached centuries ago through painstaking observation of their own bodies and the world around them.

Their research confirmed that people responded in very different ways to similar events and environments. What seemed to have no effect on one person could just as easily lead to serious illness in another. For example, some people could spend the day walking in the rain with no adverse effects, while some of their companions would have caught colds by nightfall.

As a result of their meticulous observations, the philosopher-scientists asked themselves: what was different about the people who were able to withstand the cold and damp which, at the same time, had the power to cause other people to suffer? Since the external conditions were the same for everyone, it was obvious that those whose health was unaffected must have some sort of invisible ability or power that enabled them to remain in good health.

We see the same phenomenon in people around us every day: even when everyone in the same group is exposed to the same virus, eats the same contaminated food, or is caught up in the same stressful situation, there are important differences between the individual reactions of each person.

The same is true of people's differing reactions to medical treatments. In all medical systems, whether conventional or complementary, it is well known that individuals respond in different ways even when they have the same diagnosis and receive the same treatment.

None of this extraordinary variety in human experience would have been surprising to the natural scientists and medical specialists of early Chinese civilization.

The patterns of energy

Our energy patterns are as unique to us as our thumbprint. They determine the way we interact with everything else in the world. The level of vitality can determine our resistance to the millions of bacteria in our environment, our reactions to accidents and injuries, and our responses to the countless mental stresses of life. The state of our energy also determines how we respond to any form of medicine we may be prescribed.

Your energy pattern can be symbolically illustrated in a form that resembles a graph. Each of the symbolic representations that follow corresponds to the recommended practices in this book.

Weak, fluctuating energy
You feel completely drained of vitality. You may have a persistent illness or you are suffering from a bug that has laid you low. You experience some form of depression.

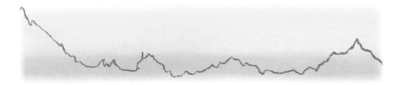

You feel tired and run down at times and then you experience a short rush of energy. You may be susceptible to colds and other short-term conditions. When you recover you feel great for a few days or even longer, then you suddenly get exhausted or sick again.

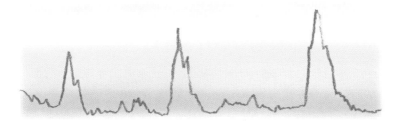

These two graphs show weak, fluctuating energy. If this is what you experience, your safest starting point will be the practices for recovering your health, found in Part Five, Returning to the Source.

Not ill, not fully well

You feel fine some days, but often you have a sense of not being well. There is nothing to go to the doctor about, but you experience periods of fatigue. You lack stamina, and are easily irritated or stressed.

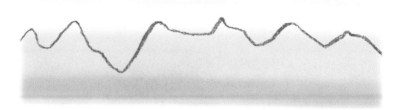

This is what we often call "normal" health. Your energy hovers around the median between high and low. Try the practices recommended in Part One, The Inner Sea.

Stronger and smoother

If you are very fit, you may find that you already have reasonably consistent levels of alertness and stamina. But there is sometimes a quality of impatience or aggression in the energy. As you follow the practices through Parts One and Two of this book, your energy pattern starts to show greater strength, but also greater calm.

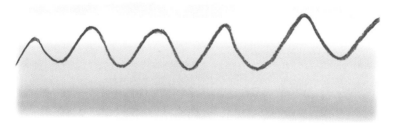

Even if you feel you can handle the practices in Parts Two and Three, which will help develop a more stable energy pattern, you are strongly advised to be sure you can accomplish the practices in Part One first.

Radiating outward

The practices in this book ultimately result in an energy pattern which is exceptionally strong. You are dynamic and rarely ill. You have a rapid recovery rate. Distress tends to be short lived.

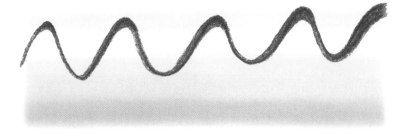

Other people sense your energy and are attracted to it. You may be able to use it to help others. Part Four, Removing the Obstacles, gives you suggestions on how you can use this exceptionally high energy to benefit yourself and others.

The wave forms

The energy patterns are shown as waves because all energy has this vibrating quality. The waves also remind us that we all experience ups and downs, good days and poor days, feel elated and get irritated, regardless of how weak or strong our energy may be.

Contemporary lifestyles are often based on a mistaken assumption that it should be possible for us to carry on from one day to the next as if nothing needed to change, as if we were perpetual motion machines. So it is important to see the whole picture presented over the next two pages, not merely as a linear progression from weakness to strength, but also as an ability to ride the waves of our ordinary, fluctuating experience of life.

This understanding of human energy has a profound effect on the meaning of the word "healing".

The Spectrum of Energy

You are weak,
feel depressed,
or are ill.

Your energy
fluctuates.
You get ill
easily.

You begin
to feel an
increase in
stamina.

HIGH ENERGY

STRONG
IMMUNITY

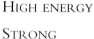

LOW ENERGY

POOR
IMMUNITY

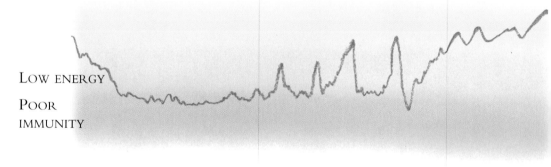

This spectrum of energy is a symbolic representation of
the way your energy develops as you progress from
being weak and ill through convalescence, normal
health and then, with the aid of the energy exercises in
this book, on to far higher levels of energy.

You have
higher levels
of energy
and alertness.

Your energy
is strong.
You can
help others.

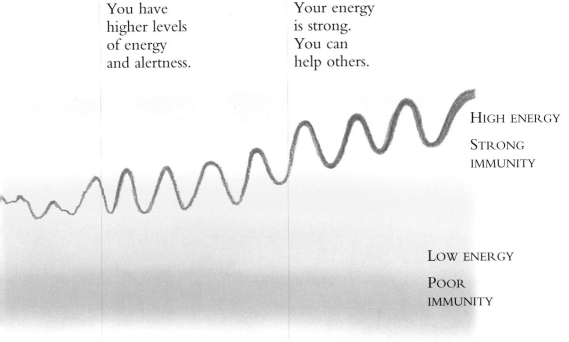

HIGH ENERGY

STRONG
IMMUNITY

LOW ENERGY

POOR
IMMUNITY

The patterns show the qualities and quantities of your energy. The quality may be erratic and fluctuating with a vibrational quality similar to a fast heart rate or it may be more even, stable and with a longer "wave pattern". The quantity is shown by the thickness of the lines – thin represents a low volume of energy which is easily diminished by over-exercise or stress. The thicker line represents the far greater volume developed by sustained Chi Kung practice.

Understanding healing

The idea of healing in Chinese health care begins with an understanding of the energy of each person. The Chinese use the character Chi, pronounced "Chee", to refer to this energy. Sometimes it is referred to as "internal energy" because it is so essential to our lives. If this energy is blocked – by a physical injury, by muscular tension, by internal obstructions, by stress – and cannot flow freely and naturally throughout your body, pain and disease will result. To heal the condition, it is necessary to remove the obstacles to the free flow of Chi and restore the natural balance of energy in your being.

This process of healing is happening spontaneously all the time. In contemporary science it is called "homeostasis"– the self-regulating power that keeps the countless activities of the body in balance with each other. The practices in this book support that process and enable your Chi to deal automatically with a range of conditions which might otherwise require external treatment.

Similarly, if your energy level is low, you need to find ways to build up your inner strength. You may not have the advanced symptoms of a conventional disease, but any imbalance or depletion of your body's energy is a pre-condition which will almost certainly later manifest as illness.

For this reason, Chinese medicine places great emphasis on preventive health care. Caring for your energy is part of a constant process of healing.

This emphasis on the importance of internal energy is also true when you are being treated for an illness or injury. Our internal energy functions like a carrier wave or a waterway. We need a good, strong current so that the full benefits of treatment are distributed throughout our entire system. In order to recover fully, therefore, we need to be sure that, at the same time as we are receiving treatment and medication, we are doing everything possible to strengthen the carrier wave of our energy.

Having a healthy understanding of the way our energy works is important. We are constantly being sold tablets to smooth out all the ups and downs of our lives. Yet health often has more in common with a wave of energy than a straight line. What is frequently treated as a "disorder" may in fact be simply the body's natural self-regulation. Suppressing the symptoms of this reaction may offer short-term relief, but may be disrupting the underlying healing process already taking place.

Caring for yourself

One of the most important principles in Chinese medicine is that each person can take responsibility for their own health. Of course, babies need to be looked after, and so do the very ill and the dying. But often the very best care we can give even in these situations is to nurture the natural processes taking place in the person's life.

We can apply this profound philosophy in our daily lives. It is a mistake to think that we can find health by relying solely on outside care. The greatest surgeons and pharmacists all tell us that the success of any treatment depends not only on the skill of the medical specialist, but also on the behaviour of the patient, including their will to recover. The decisive role each person plays in their own health has been a central feature of Chinese health care from the earliest days. This culture of personal responsibility includes regular maintenance of each individual's energy levels.

Throughout the Chinese-speaking world, countless people, from the very young to the very old, begin their day attending to their health. You see them everywhere in the parks and gardens, performing a remarkable variety of movements – all designed to cultivate their internal energy.

The form of this type of exercise, as you will see from the practices presented in this book, is not the sort of punishing activity often associated with fitness exercise in the West.

The healing and strengthening exercises in this book are gentle. They are practised slowly and calmly. Some practices involve no movement at all. You simply hold a position, perhaps making slight adjustments such as raising or lowering your toes while sitting still.

On the surface, this sort of inner work appears to be almost the opposite of exercise. Yet it is through these deceptively simple methods that generations have learned to care for themselves and their families through all the stresses and strains of a lifetime.

Cultivating energy

The Chinese term for cultivating energy is *Chi Kung*. *Kung* means exercise or sweat. So *Chi Kung* literally means "internal energy exercise".

A great range of these energy development techniques have been created over the years. They include systems of movement, such as Tai Chi Chuan, and others which involve breathing exercises and visualizations.

All these systems are based on a profound understanding of the human being as a complete field of energy. Unlike certain medical models that make a sharp distinction between the body and the mind, the Chinese perception of the human being is of an integrated energy field. This field, like a miniature cosmos, embraces every particle in our body, every flicker of our nervous system and every thought and emotion.

The healing effect

Once every person is understood to be an entire field of energy, the idea of "energy exercise" takes on a deeper meaning. We are practising something that affects our entire being.

Because of their total approach, the exercises in this book have a holistic effect on each person, regardless of the state of their health. They can be used by those who are extremely weak, perhaps seriously ill or recuperating from an illness or operation. They will address not only the person's physical condition, but also the accompanying mental and emotional states which need to be strengthened if they are to return to full strength.

This approach to healing is very personal. The movements and the positions, particularly in the early stages of practice, are standard. But the way they affect each person varies according to their individual needs and capacity.

Whether you are an office worker, manager, manual labourer, homemaker or performer, the long-term results of regular training will be unmistakable. If your internal organs are functioning harmoniously, your health will benefit and you will have high tolerance for stress. If you are relaxed under pressure, you will be more productive. Regular practice will ensure that your power will be directed by a mind that is increasingly alert and sensitive.

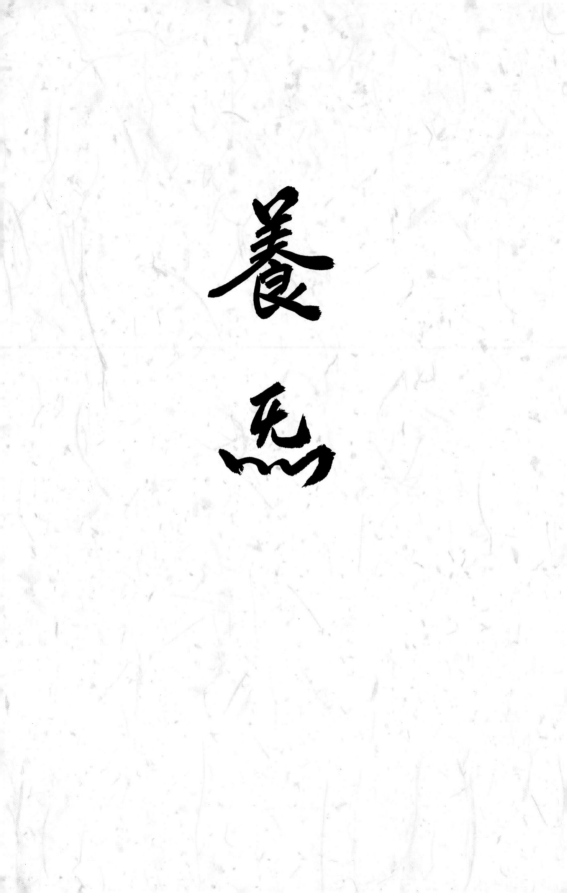

養鳥

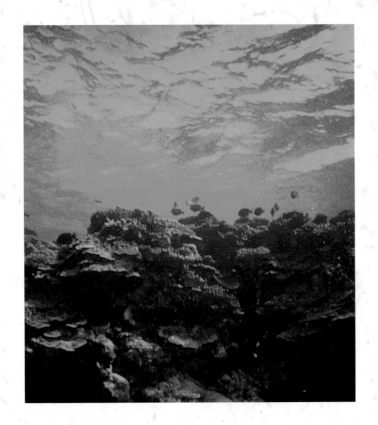

PART ONE

THE
INNER
SEA
Sustaining your Health

Introduction

*Those who disobey the laws of the universe
will give rise to calamities and visitations,
while those who follow the laws of the universe
remain free from dangerous illness.*

THE YELLOW EMPEROR'S CLASSIC
OF INTERNAL MEDICINE

Everyday life is full of unease. Often we wake up
feeling unslept. We drag ourselves out of bed
reluctantly and are surrounded by the hassles of family
life, getting ready for work or school. We have a rushed
breakfast, hearing the latest news on the radio or TV.
Then off into the rush hour or on to the treadmill of
housework. Lunch is often a frantic affair, followed by a
tiring afternoon. The tension lets up a little in the
evening sometimes, but not always. Sometimes we push
ourselves late into the night.

Some people try to relax by flopping in front of the TV
or looking for oblivion through various addictions.
Others continue to drive themselves in the pursuit of
physical fitness. If we manage to keep going like this,
with only a few bouts of flu or the occasional cold, we
call ourselves healthy.

But underneath the dynamic activity, and even the
periods of apparent relaxation, there is constant anxiety.
It affects every aspect of our being, from our heart and
lungs right through to our bones and muscles. We
know we may not be seeing a doctor, but we know
we are far from well.

Trapped in this indeterminate state of unease, we are
slowly but surely wearing ourselves out. It gets harder
and harder to recover our full strength. Our emotions
take their toll on us and we find it harder to bounce
back after being irritated or shocked.

This is the condition of "not ill, not fully well" described on page 12. Its energy pattern looks like this:

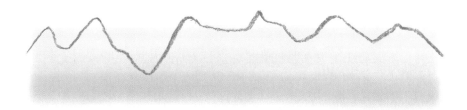

In reality this state is the fertile breeding ground for serious ill health. In Traditional Chinese Medicine, it is anxiety and stress which subtly silt up the energy pathways within the body until the flow of Chi is cut off. The inner sea runs dry. When that nourishment ceases to bathe any part of the organism, cells die and organs start to wither.

The good news is that this debilitating process can be reversed through the age-old methods of relaxation and the natural cultivation of energy to which you are introduced in this part of the book. The core practice is known as Zhan Zhuang (pronounced "Jam Jong"), which literally means "Standing Like a Tree".

The techniques are simple, but the wisdom which has refined them over the centuries is profound. They are the essential entry point for the advanced practices presented later in the book.

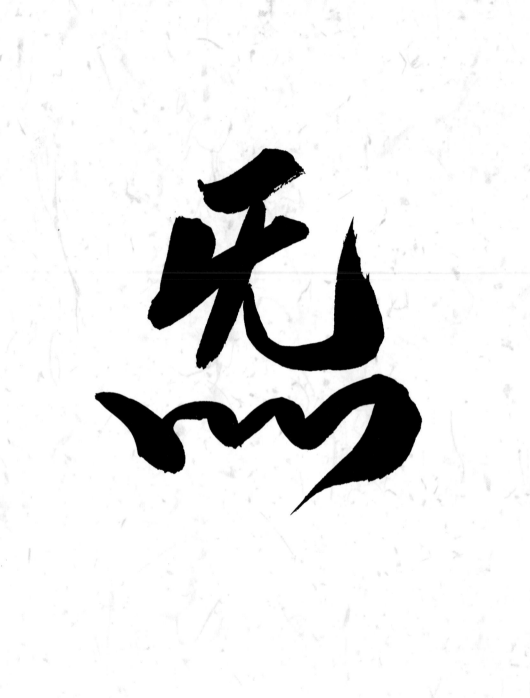

Chi

Chi is the invisible life force of the universe. It is the essence of our existence. "In order to do anything in this life, we must first have energy," wrote the ancient Chinese philosopher Guan Tse.

The Chinese character for Chi, often used by officials in contemporary China and frequently seen in books sold in the West, conveys the meaning of "breath" or "air". Hence the common mistake that Chi Kung is simply a set of breathing exercises. Using this character leads to an even more unfortunate misunderstanding: it gives the impression that Chi is something external to us.

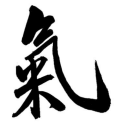

The original character used by the ancient scholars and Chi Kung masters is shown on the facing page. It conveys the true nature of Chi, and hence the inner meaning of Chi Kung.

The character has two elements. On top is a square resembling a container or a pot with a handle.

Underneath the container are four strokes. They rise upwards, representing fire.

Taken together, the image is one of a container placed over a fire, like an iron pot in which water is being brought to the boil over an open flame.

As the water is heated, it gradually begins to manifest a more active quality. It remains water, but we see movement within it. Slowly, as it heats up, a subtle vapour begins to rise from the liquid. Eventually, intense energy is released from its depths in the form of bubbles which rise through the liquid and burst into the atmosphere.

This calligraphy is itself a metaphor for the powerful transformation of your own internal energy that will result from the practices in this book.

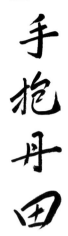

Gathering your Chi

Each human life forms around a central point. The tiny cells begin to multiply around the area where the fetus is directly connected to the mother's womb.

Deep in the womb, this early growth is invisible. Within that silent environment, the life force manifests as a warm and moist plasma, abundant with fertility.

The point of connection becomes our umbilical cord, sustaining the vital exchange between mother and baby. Once cut, the cells reform to create the newborn's navel, or belly button. We tend to forget this history as we grow, but it is of supreme importance in the medical model on which Chinese medicine is based.

Associated with your navel is the Sea of Chi, called in Chinese Tan Tien (pronounced "Dan Dyen"). It lies 3 cm (1.25 in) below your navel, one-third of the way into your body. It is the reservoir of your Chi – just as it was in the womb.

The first step in the practice of The Way of Healing is to ensure that this inner reservoir is replenished. The method for doing this is simply to spend some time "gathering your chi" by folding your hands calmly over your Tan Tien.

Start by standing in a relaxed, upright position. Your feet should be placed so that they are shoulder width apart, with the toes pointing forward.

Rest the side of your right thumb over your navel so that the rest of your hand naturally falls into place over your lower abdomen. Then place your left hand comfortably on top of your right.

You can lower your eyelids, but keep your eyes open. Breathe naturally.

Practice standing for up to two minutes at a time. Slowly build up to five minutes.

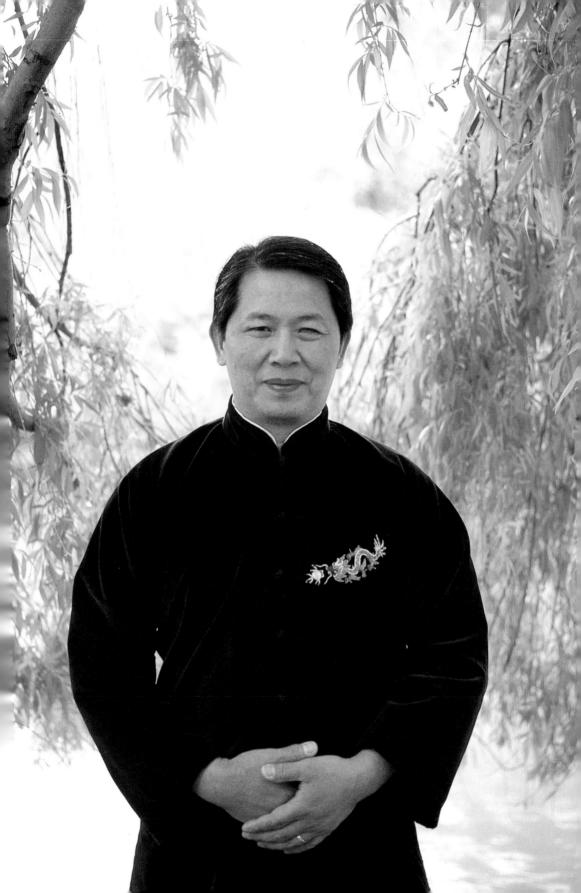

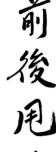

Arousing your Chi

This deceptively simple exercise starts to move your Chi outwards from its reservoir in your abdomen all the way to your finger tips. You do it in a very relaxed way, gently swinging your arms backwards and forwards, like a pendulum.

Stand still with your feet facing forward, shoulder–width apart.

Look straight forward with your head held erect. Tuck your chin very slightly in so that your head is neither slumped forward nor tilted backward. Relax your shoulders and let your hands hang loosely by your sides.

Imagine that you are about to sit down on a stool behind you. Let your backside relax and gently lower yourself down about 2 cm (1 in). This naturally causes your knees to bend slightly, but not to protrude forward over your toes. Adjust your position so that your weight is spread evenly over your feet.

1. Swing both your arms loosely forwards, as if the back of your hands were leading the motion. Your hands come up to a point level with your chest, but not higher than your shoulders. Your fingers are gently spread apart.

2. Swing your arms back until they naturally stop. Keep them slightly away from your body, not closing in behind your back.

Then let the natural momentum of the swing carry them forward again. Build up a spontaneous and rapid swing, as if you were flinging your fingers outwards and immediately pulling them back within a second.

Begin with 50 complete swings, trying to keep your body stable. Then progress up to 200.

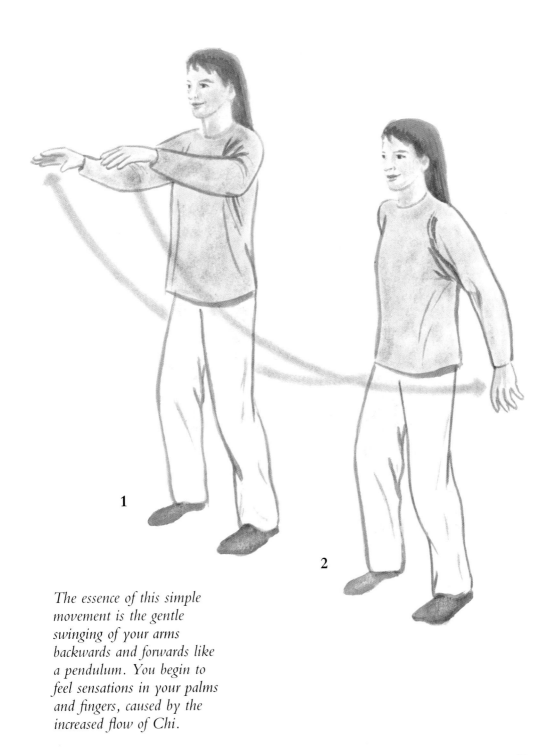

1

2

The essence of this simple movement is the gentle swinging of your arms backwards and forwards like a pendulum. You begin to feel sensations in your palms and fingers, caused by the increased flow of Chi.

Increasing your Inner Warmth

This exercise is based on one of the many ways we
naturally warm ourselves. Many people spontaneously
slap themselves to get warm. In this exercise, you slap
the outer side of your thighs, which stimulates the
movement of warming Chi as it flows through the
energy pathways up the outer side of your leg.

Stand with your feet facing forward, shoulder-width
apart. Unlock your knees so that they relax, but do not
protrude forward. Check that your weight is evenly
spread over both your feet.

Relax your upper body. Make sure that your shoulders
are free from tension so that your arms can hang loosely
by your sides.

Look straight forward with a calm gaze.

Begin slapping the outside of your thighs with the
relaxed palms of your hands.

Breathe naturally as you do this.

Begin with 30 slaps and build up if you feel comfortable
and able to continue. Do this with a comfortable pace
in your own time – not too quickly, not too slowly.
The slaps should be firm, but not too hard. Stop when
you feel you have done enough, and don't push yourself
to the point where your thighs or palms hurt.

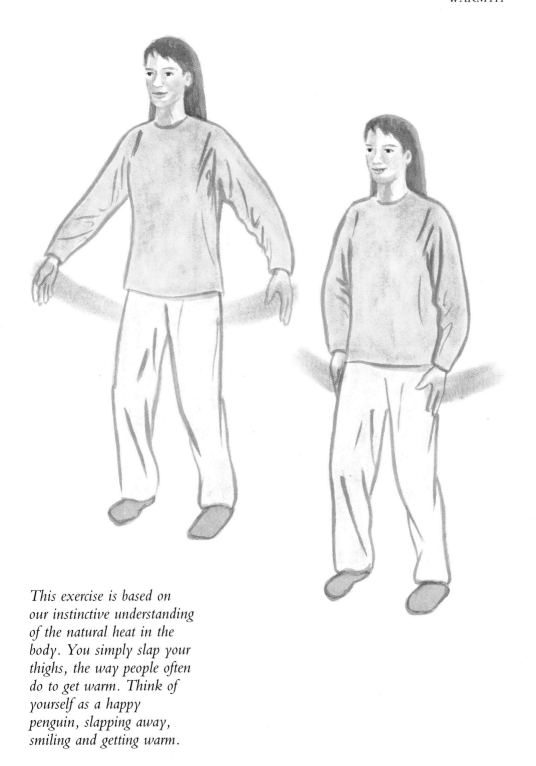

This exercise is based on our instinctive understanding of the natural heat in the body. You simply slap your thighs, the way people often do to get warm. Think of yourself as a happy penguin, slapping away, smiling and getting warm.

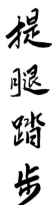

Raising your Internal Power

This exercise uses your shifting body weight to pump your Chi through your body. This action is triggered by the changing pressure on the nerve endings and acupuncture points in the soles of your feet.

Stand with your feet facing forward, shoulder-width apart. Place your hands calmly beside you. Relax your entire upper body. Look straight ahead.

1. Shift your weight on to your left foot. Imagine that all your weight sinks down through the left side of your body, down through the sole of your foot, into the ground.

2. When you feel you have allowed your weight to sink fully down through your foot, gently lift your right foot until your knee is level with your hip.

As you lift your leg, breathe in.

Lift your leg so that there is a right angle between your calf and your thigh. This will keep the whole of your leg out in front of your body, not tucking under towards your back.

Lift your toes, so the sole of your foot is parallel to the floor, not dropping downward.

Then, as your breathe out, gently lower your right foot back down to the ground.

3. Now shift your weight over to your right foot.

4. Gently lift and lower your left leg in the same way. Begin with 6 alternate liftings and lowerings and build up to 12.

Then stand still with your weight evenly spread over both feet. Rest in that position for one minute.

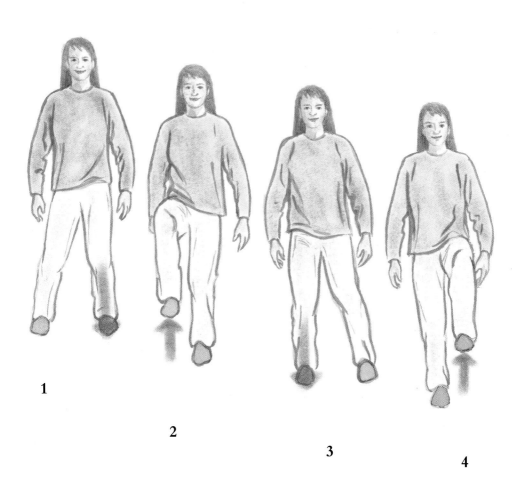

1

2

3

4

*This gentle exercise resembles
"marking time", raising each leg in
front and placing it back down. As
you change legs, give your full
attention each time first to establishing
your balance on the sole of the foot
that supports your weight. Feel the
powerful contact you make with the
solidity of the earth below.*

The Position of Primal Energy

Once you have completed the three movement exercises on the previous pages, your body will be sufficiently warmed up to allow you to experience the effects of increased Chi without harming yourself. It is therefore extremely important to complete the previous exercises before proceeding to this stage.

You begin with the first of the ancient Chinese Chi Kung postures. This stationary position is known in Chinese as Wu Chi, the position of primal energy.

If you are able to practise outside, this is best. You can do all the preceding exercises first and then stand in Wu Chi. Try to find a place where you can face a large tree, with the sun on your back. Don't stand outside in the rain and fog.

Some people find it difficult to do this practice outdoors. In that case, practise indoors. Try to use a relatively quiet room. A recording of flowing instrumental music may help. If possible, open a window to ensure a current of fresh air.

The key points of the posture are given on the facing page. Pages 36–7 will help ensure that you are correctly aligned between the energies of earth and space. The mental work that accompanies this is described on pages 38–9.

When you start, even very short periods can seem endless. Since we rarely spend any time in stillness, the first experience can come as a shock. Begin for a minute or two, and then progress from there until you are able to hold the posture for ten minutes.

Do not worry about how long it takes you to reach this length of time. Do not push yourself beyond your capacity. When you feel the need to stop, place your hands over your Tan Tien (see pages 26–7) for a short period before moving.

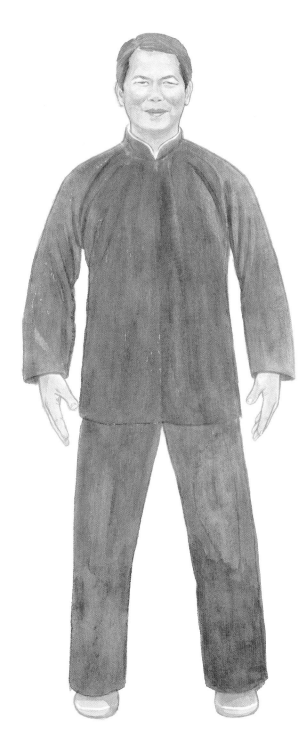

1. *Stand still with your feet shoulder width apart. Relax your knees.*

2. *Let your belly and hips relax.*

3. *Sightly sink your chest inward. Let your shoulders naturally ease downward.*

4. *Let your arms hang loosely by your sides. Your fingers should be slightly apart, naturally curved.*

5. *Lower your chin a little and relax your neck.*

6. *Look forward and slightly downward.*

7. *Breathe calmly through your nose.*

Finding your Centre

Tension and illness often cause us to be off-centre. Over the years we become accustomed to holding our bodies in slightly crooked or tilted postures. The result is that when we stand straight we feel awkward. That is why it is so important to check that you are standing vertically in this exercise. As you practise, your inner gyroscope will adjust to the correct, healthy posture.

You should be standing straight. Check that you are evenly balanced between your feet without leaning to one side, so that the centre line of your body is vertical. Your Tan Tien, shown by the red dot on the facing page below the figure's navel, is in line with the central point at the top of your head and directly over the central line between your feet.

Your weight should be spread evenly on the soles of your feet. Make sure that you are not leaning forwards or backwards.

Relax your knees. You can check if they are relaxed by locking them tightly and then letting the muscles naturally unlock. As you can see from the drawings on the facing page, your knees do not protrude forward over your toes.

As you stand, feel that the distribution of weight in your body is like that of a pyramid. Your feet are the base. Your head is the peak. The base, spread firmly on the earth, is wide, dark and heavy. The peak, pointing towards the sky, is lofty, radiant and light.

In this relaxed, natural stance the feeling of heaviness in your feet is the signal that you are making contact with the earth's energy. The lighter sensation in the area of your head is your own awareness of contact with the energy of space.

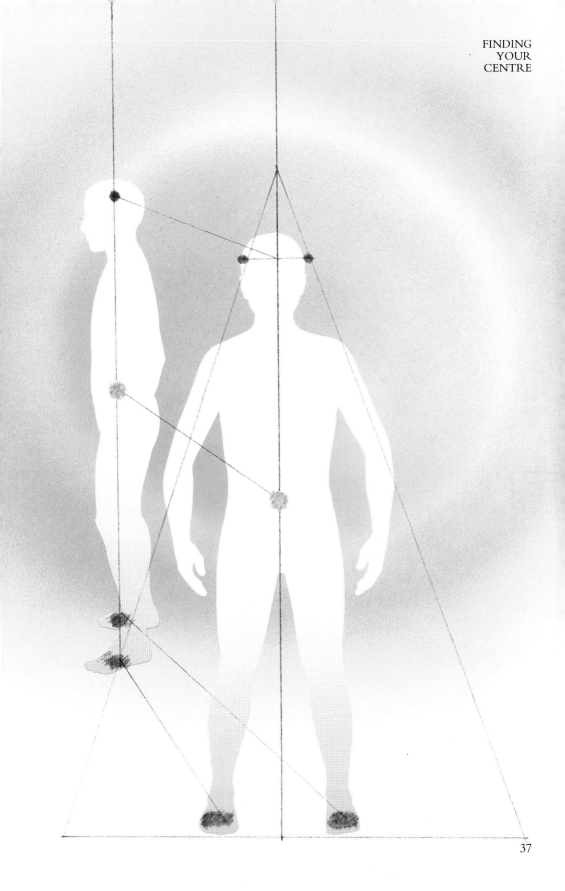

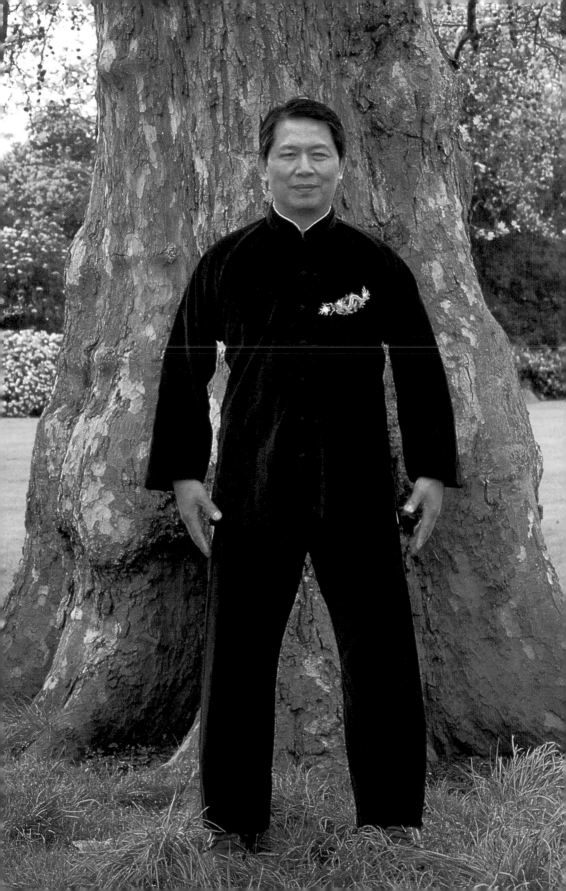

Calming the Spirit

Chi Kung calms your nervous system. As you stand in Wu Chi, follow this inner relaxation sequence.

First, take your mind to the area around your eyes. Let go of any tension you may be holding in the skin or muscles.

Then, take your mind to your jawbone and release any tension there.

Let this feeling of relaxation flow down both sides of your neck like a warm, golden liquid.

Let it flow over your right shoulder. Allow your arm to slide downward. When you feel it hanging loosely like a weight by your side, do the same with your left shoulder and arm.

Breathe out so that your chest sinks inward a little and your shoulders curve slightly forward.

Imagine your back is caked in thick mud. A fresh waterfall begins to cascade down your back, washing away all traces of the mud. It flows down over your buttocks, releasing any tension held in your hips.

Feel your feet bearing the full weight of your body. You are rooted to the earth.

Then take your attention to the very top of your head. Imagine a fine golden thread supporting you, stretching up into the heavens. You feel a slight upward lift in the body.

You rest in stillness, aware of the heaviness in the soles of your feet and the lightness at the top of your head.

The Two Powers

There are three stages to practising Wu Chi correctly. First, you have to work on your stance and the correct alignment of your body. This starts to open up your inner energy pathways (see Finding your Centre on pages 36–7). Second, you need to practise relaxing, working quietly and carefully down your body through all the muscle groups to release accumulated tension (see Calming your Spirit on pages 38–9).

Third, to experience the full healing power of Chi Kung, you need to have in your mind a clear vision of what is happening to you. In classical Chinese this would be called a vision of Heaven and Earth. In many ways, it is exactly the same portrait of the cosmos as that now revealed by the most sophisticated discoveries of contemporary scientists.

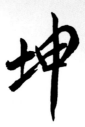

Earth

You are standing upright on Earth. It is a sphere of energy blessed with extraordinary fertility. The soil, water and atmosphere have sustained countless life forms since the dawn of nature. From microscopic organisms to the great mammals, there seems to be no limit to the number or variety of living beings. Yet the abundance of the biosphere is only the merest fraction of the earth's energy. Even greater is the hidden power of the vast sea of fire constantly burning beneath the earth's crust. This is the living entity on which you rest and feed as you make your journey through space.

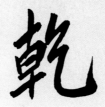

Heaven

With each new breakthrough in the exploration of space, the detectable universe expands. The images sent back to our listening posts on the earth reveal a universe whose limits are unknown. We see wonders that are increasingly vast and extraordinarily intricate. They are spellbinding in their beauty. It is out of this immense, luminous field that we emerge. Our entire existence is based on its incalculable energy. As you stand in Wu Chi, properly aligned and deeply relaxed, you begin to open more and more to this radiating power that surrounds you.

鬆
肩
提
抱

The Full Belly

The healing power of Chi Kung works deep within the body. As you slowly open up to the energies of Heaven and Earth, allow nature to take its course and avoid rushing ahead too quickly.

Before moving on to this next standing position you should have developed a regular routine of Gathering your Chi (pages 26–7) for up to five minutes, followed by the three exercises – Arousing your Chi (pages 28–9), Increasing your Inner Warmth (pages 30–1) and Raising your Internal Power (pages 32–3) – and then standing in the Wu Chi position (pages 34–5) for at least 10 minutes.

This next posture, the Full Belly, helps your spine decompress. As you hold the slightly lower position, the extra work done by your leg muscles stimulates the circulation of blood throughout your body.

To practise this posture, begin by standing in Wu Chi. Your feet should be shoulder-width apart with your toes pointing forwards.

Lower your bottom slightly, about 2 cm (1 in), as if you were about to sit down. This will cause your knees to bend slightly, but make sure they do not come forward over your toes. Feel your lower back relaxing, as if you were resting on an invisible stool.

Completely relax your belly so that it expands naturally outward. Imagine it is extending beyond your body – bring both your hands up in front of your abdomen as if you were holding them around the fullness that extends beyond your body.

You may find it easier to try imagining that your hands are holding a large golden sphere in front of your belly. As you do this, relax your palms. Feel that they are on the sides of the sphere. Rather than being turned sharply upwards, they are gently curved as if following the smooth arc of the surface.

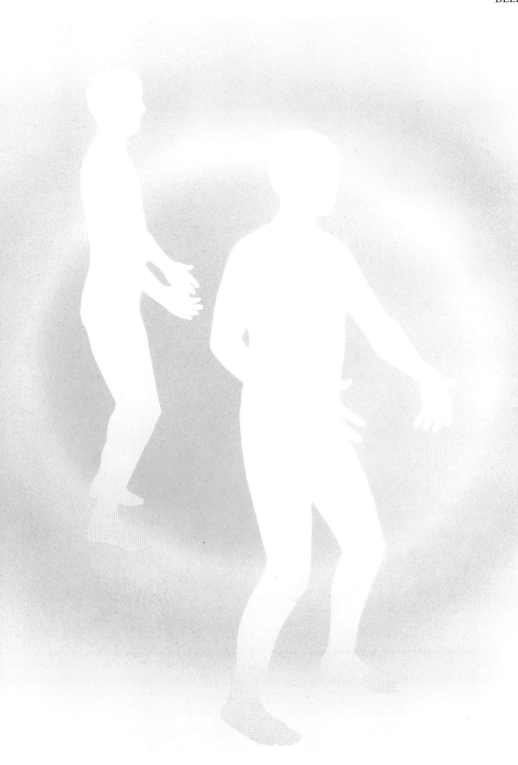

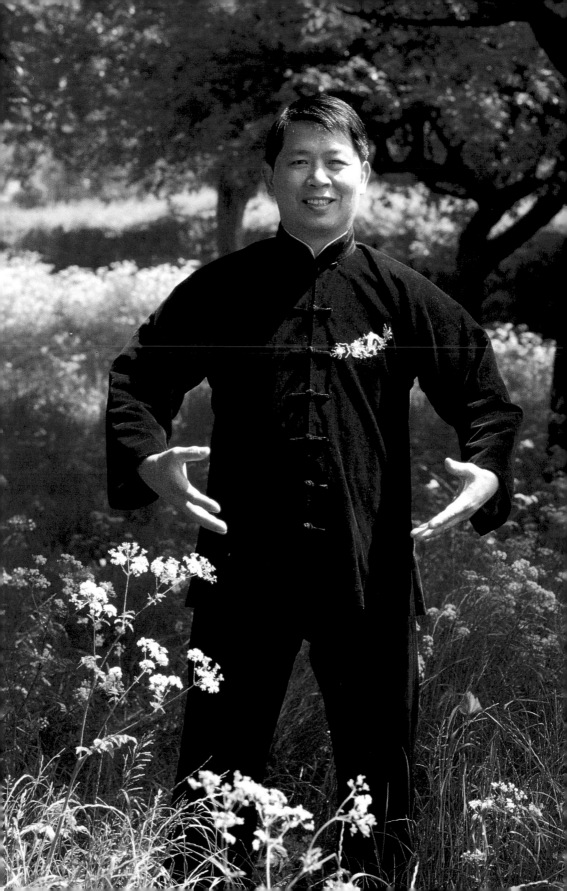

鬆
肩
提
抱

After a delicious meal you feel a certain secret pleasure in the warmth and fullness of your belly. This is not the same sensation that you get if you overeat. It is the natural feeling of inner happiness which causes you to become aware of the relaxed expansiveness in the whole area of your hips, pelvis, lower back and abdomen. If you allow yourself to explore those sensations, you discover a delightful feeling, as if you were being gently warmed from within.

This is the sensation that gradually develops when you stand holding the Full Belly, with your hands just beyond your lower abdomen. To do this properly, you need to give permission to all the muscles in your belly to relax.

It may help you to think of the figure of The Laughing Buddha, the classical figure that you often see in Chinese shops, with a broad smile and a rotund belly. His belly is not considered fat, but rather filled with energy. In the legends surrounding this figure, it is said that his Chi was so powerful that when he lay down to sleep by the roadside, his radiant energy would melt falling snowflakes before they even touched his body.

When holding the Full Belly, many people tend to hunch their shoulders and to strain their chest muscles as they hold their arms in front. One way to eliminate this unnecessary tension is to imagine that there is a strap running around behind your neck and stretching down to your wrists. The strap takes all the weight of your arms and, at the same time, has the effect of lowering your shoulders and relaxing your chest.

Try holding this position for five minutes. Then return to Wu Chi for a couple of minutes. Finish by Gathering your Chi (pages 26–7) for a final minute or two.

As you become more familiar with relaxing in this position, extend your practice so that you are able to hold this posture for up to 10 minutes.

行為

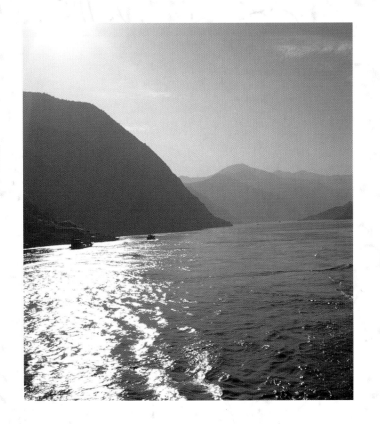

PART TWO

THE
GREAT
RIVER

Increasing your Energy

Introduction

People are born gentle and weak.
At their death they are hard and stiff.
Green plants are tender and filled with sap.
At their death they are withered and dry.
Therefore the stiff and unbending is the disciple of death.
The gentle and yielding is the disciple of life.

LAO TSE

The natural tendency of Chi is to move. It is like the current of a river. When the current is weak, the water will stagnate. In Traditional Chinese Medicine, many common conditions are said to result from Stagnant Chi – coldness, congestion, stiffness and aching joints.

Using the practices in this book, we are able to transform any underlying patterns of Stagnant Chi and restore the natural, strong flow of the energy. This change corresponds to the pattern, "Stronger and Smoother", described in the Introduction on page 12.

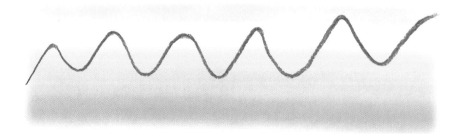

To keep the Chi flowing throughout the body, many different exercises have been developed over the years. Perhaps the best known is Tai Chi – the slow, gentle movement system that is widespread throughout the Chinese-speaking world.

In this part of the book you are introduced to some of the most fundamental Tai Chi movements, which you find in the famous schools and styles of Tai Chi.

You should start to practise these movements once you have reached the point where you can comfortably sustain the practices to which you were introduced in Part One of this book. Especially if your energy levels have been low, you need to increase the volume of Chi stored in your internal reservoir (the Tan Tien) and practise the opening positions of Zhan Zhuang. This will give you the strength to continue on your path of healing. Without these energy reserves your Tai Chi will be weak and often empty.

When you start to work with the movement exercises in this part of the book, you should keep up your regular Zhan Zhuang training. You should have reached the point where you can stand in Wu Chi for at least ten minutes. Your daily routine should begin with that and then include the various Tai Chi movements that you are learning.

It is best to learn one movement at a time. Follow the instructions carefully. Check your own movements in a mirror or with a friend. Try to be as precise as possible. When you become familiar with the movement, aim to make it as gracefully as possible, without any breaks or jerks in the flowing motion.

The combination of this movement work with your Zhan Zhuang training means that you will gradually develop a powerful inner sensation of stability and stillness while moving calmly and effortlessly like a great river.

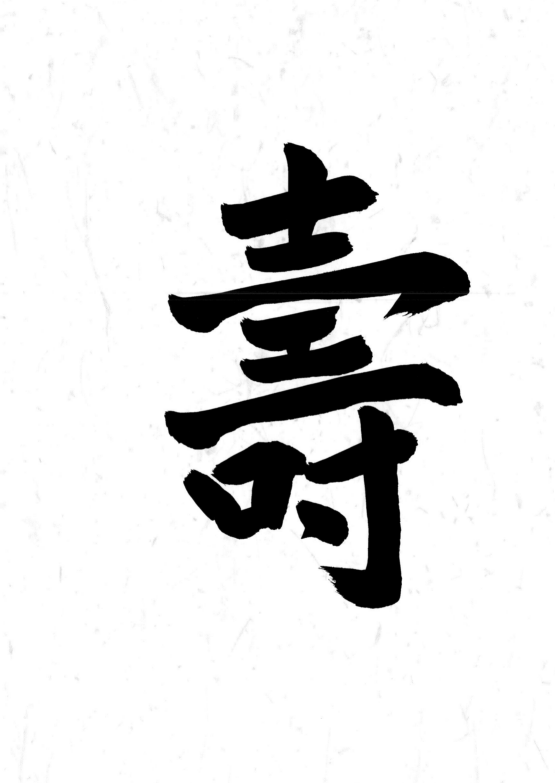

Long Life

The Chinese character on the facing page means
longevity. In some cultures, people tend to picture
a long life as a single line from birth through maturity
to death. The classical Chinese ideogram is strikingly
different.

In the upper part of the character, the energy alternates
between long, broad strokes and shorter, compressed,
brush movements just as the energy of the sea expresses
itself in alternating waves of expansion and recoil.

Embodied in this representation of a long life is a vision
of health based not upon a selective notion of fitness,
but on the entire fabric of a lifetime, including those
episodes we call illness.

At the very base of the character is a simple downward
stroke. The entire weight of the ideogram rests upon it.
This is the brush stroke for the human hand, symbol-
izing a person bearing the pressure of a lifetime.

Interestingly, the character is not symmetrically
balanced. It is an ancient view, yet astonishingly
contemporary. Among the most recent scientific
theories is a view that sees life as naturally unbalanced,
a constant interchange of stillness and motion,
expressing the immense, perpetually changing energy
of the universe.

Within this constant flow of energy, the fully matured
person is able to stand, stable and rooted, at one with all
life's events.

Thus, as the Taoist sage Chuang-tse approached death,
he restrained his distraught disciples who wanted to give
him a grand funeral. He smiled: "Heaven and Earth will
be my coffin. The sun and moon will be the jade
symbols hanging by my sides. All the planets and
constellations will shine around me like jewels. What
more could I need? Everything has already been taken
care of."

Drawing Silk from the Cocoon

This graceful movement stretches back to a time when threads of raw silk were slowly unreeled by hand from the cocoons of silk worms. To withdraw the long filaments unbroken, a relaxed, continuous motion was needed that was neither too limp nor too strong. The following silk-reeling exercise creates a state of powerful relaxation in which the mind remains alert and stimulates the flow of Chi out to the finger tips.

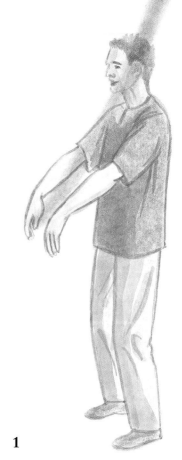

1. Stand still with your feet facing forward, shoulder-width apart. Relax your entire body, following the Calming the Spirit sequence on page 39. After you have completed the relaxation sequence, imagine that you are drawing out the silk fibres from the cocoons of silk worms. Each fingertip pulls a thread from a cocoon. The movement must be smooth, yet firm, so that the silk continuously unfolds but never breaks.

Slightly spread your fingers and raise them gently in front of you, with your finger tips naturally angled downward. Keep your shoulders and arms as relaxed as possible. Gently breathe in with the slow upward motion.

1

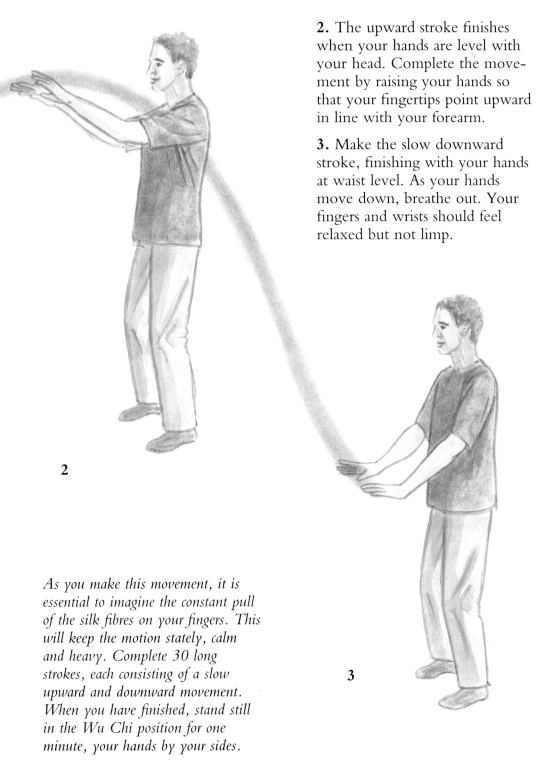

2. The upward stroke finishes when your hands are level with your head. Complete the movement by raising your hands so that your fingertips point upward in line with your forearm.

3. Make the slow downward stroke, finishing with your hands at waist level. As your hands move down, breathe out. Your fingers and wrists should feel relaxed but not limp.

2

As you make this movement, it is essential to imagine the constant pull of the silk fibres on your fingers. This will keep the motion stately, calm and heavy. Complete 30 long strokes, each consisting of a slow upward and downward movement. When you have finished, stand still in the Wu Chi position for one minute, your hands by your sides.

3

Rolling the Golden Sphere

This movement helps circulate your energy by setting up a continuous circuit between your hands and the Sea of Chi in your Tan Tien. The slow circular movement not only stimulates the flow of Chi, but the momentum it generates increases the level of Chi itself. As you work with this exercise, you will gradually begin to feel sensations of warmth and elasticity radiating between your palms.

Stand in Wu Chi with your knees slightly bent. Place your hands in front of your belly with your palms facing each other. Imagine you are holding a large sphere of golden light or an illuminated amber globe between your hands. Your fingers are slightly spread.

1. Slowly make a circle with the imaginary sphere as if you were rolling it in a smooth circle up from your belly in the direction of your chest. Continue the circle outwards, away from you.

2. Complete the circle by bringing the sphere downward, in toward your belly. Keep your elbows loosely bent so that they move naturally with the movement of your hands.

Breathe out as the sphere circles up and outward. Breathe in as it comes down and in toward your belly.

Make a minimum of 10 of these circles and up to 30 if you want.

Now, reverse the direction in which you are rolling the illuminated sphere. Breathe out as your hands move outward, away from your body. Breathe in as your hands come in toward your belly.

Repeat a minimum of 10 circles and up to 30 in this reverse direction.

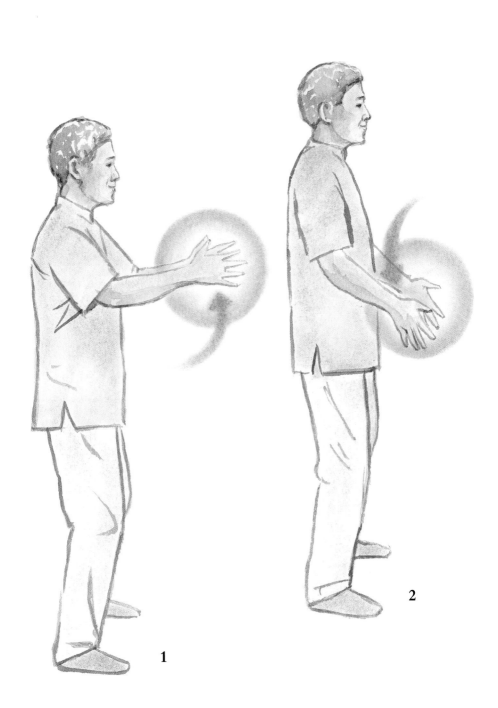

1

2

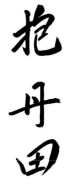

Rotating the Golden Sphere

This movement makes use of the power in your arms as a way of increasing the energy that is built up between your hands while turning the imaginary golden sphere. It is important to keep your attention on the palms of your hands, imagining the glowing golden sphere between them. This becomes the focal point for the increase of energy.

Standing in Wu Chi with your knees slightly bent, hold your hands a comfortable distance in front of you, level with the middle of your torso. Your palms face each other. Your shoulders are relaxed.

1. Visualize a golden sphere, like a glowing globe being held between your two hands. You imagine that it is warm and comfortable to touch. Your fingers should be gently spread.

2. Rotate the imaginary sphere so that your right hand comes on top and your left hand ends up underneath. Make sure that there is lots of space under your armpits and around your elbows as you make this movement. Don't hunch your shoulders. All the joints from your shoulders to your wrists and fingers should feel relaxed as your move.

3. Then rotate the sphere the other way, so that your left hand comes back up on top and your right had goes underneath.

There is no special breathing for this exercise: breathe naturally.

Make a minimum of 10 turnings of the sphere and up to 30 or more, if you are comfortable.

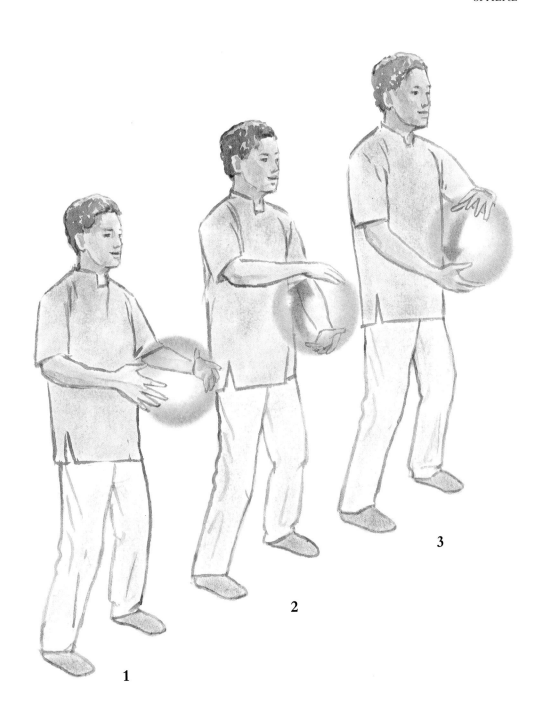

1

2

3

Looking Back at the Moon

推窗望月

This exercise extends the flow of energy through your entire body, from the soles of your feet right out to the tips of your fingers. It opens up the energy pathways in the spine and helps relieve muscular tension all along the vital energy circuits that run up the backs of the legs, through the back and along the arms. It is not advised for women during pregnancy.

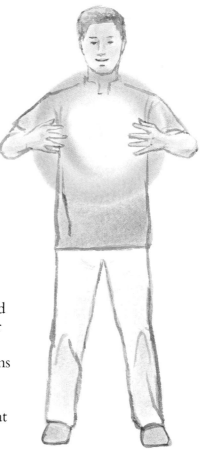

1. Stand with your feet facing forward, shoulder-width apart. Relax your knees. Your weight should be evenly distributed over both feet. Face forward. Raise your arms as if they were embracing a large balloon in front of your chest. Your palms curve in towards your body, level with your chest. Your fingers are spread apart to allow space between them. Ensure that there is plenty of air under your armpits and around your elbows. Relax your shoulders.

1

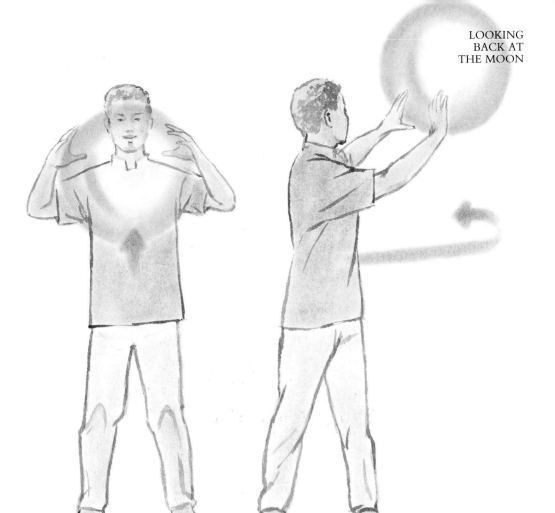

2. Raise the imaginary balloon in front of you so that your hands are just above the level of your shoulders.

3. Slowly turn your whole upper body and waist around to the left, keeping your arms and feet in position. Breathe out as you turn. Turn as far as possible without causing yourself discomfort and turn your hands outward so that both palms face away from you. Hold the position for one second.

Then slowly turn back to the front, lowering the balloon to chest level. Breathe in as you do this. As you complete the movement, turn your hands so that your palms again face your body. Face the front for one second. Repeat six times, alternating to either side.

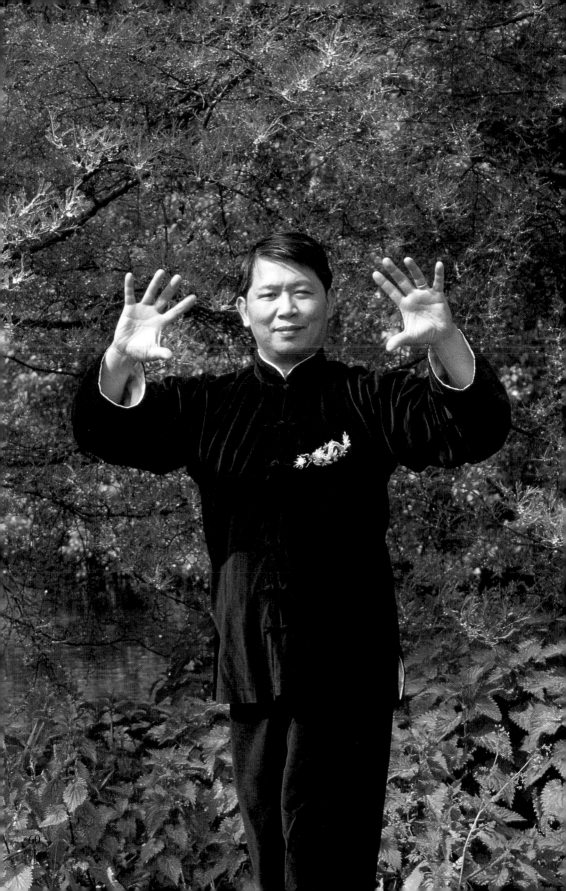

推
窗
望
月

Looking Back at the Moon is part of a set of movements known in Chinese as "The Eight Pieces of
Brocade". It was developed by the renowned 12th-
century General Yeuh Fei, whose army was never
defeated in battle. Looking Back at the Moon is one of
the most potent of the eight exercises. It stimulates the
vital power of your kidneys and entire nervous system.

As you perform the movements to each side, it is
important to maintain a solid connection with the earth.
Be sure to keep both feet flat on the floor. Don't lift
your heels as you turn. When you have turned around
as fully as possible, gently press your feet down into the
floor. Then relax and turn around towards the front.

Use your hips and waist to make the turn to each side.
Your upper body moves naturally around as a result. As
the picture on the facing page shows, the alignment of
your head, arms and hands remains constant.

Make six turns altogether, alternately turning to the left
and right. Remember to breathe out as you turn
towards the back. Pause for one second at the end of
the turn. Then breathe in as you return to face the
front. Pause and breathe naturally before starting the
turn to the other side.

At the end, return to face the front, lower your hands
to the sides and stand still for a minute to allow the full
effect of the exercise to flow through you.

Waving Hands like Clouds

This classical movement is marvellous for synchronizing your mental and physical being. It leaves you calm and refreshed. It moves your Chi throughout your entire system, and is often recommended as a way of dealing with powerful sudden stresses, including fits of anger.

The essence of the movement is to move your hands and arms in two lazy, large circles, each flowing outward to the sides, away from the centre of your body.

To begin with, stand with your feet shoulder-width apart, feet facing forward. Your knees should be slightly bent and your belly relaxed.

Raise your left hand in front of the left side of your chest and position your right hand in front of the right side of your belly. Gently open your hands so there is space between each of the fingers.

Relax your shoulders. Make sure you leave lots of space under your armpits and elbows. There should also be ample space between your palms and your body.

Start to move your left hand away to the side, turning your palm outward as you do this. Keep your elbow and wrist relaxed.

As your left hand circles away from you, start to raise your right hand up in front of you. Your head calmly turns so that your gaze can now follow the movement of your right hand.

Each hand describes a full circle as shown on the facing page. As one slowly rises in front of you and turns away, the other is completing its downward arc.

Breathe naturally as the hands move gently and continuously. Practise doing a series of 10 synchronized circles and increase to 30 if you can.

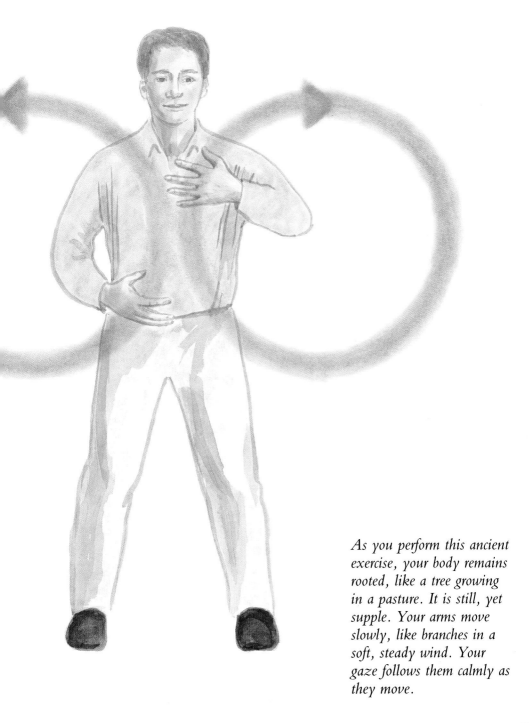

As you perform this ancient exercise, your body remains rooted, like a tree growing in a pasture. It is still, yet supple. Your arms move slowly, like branches in a soft, steady wind. Your gaze follows them calmly as they move.

To learn Waving Hands like Clouds, practise the
motion of your hands separately. When you are familiar
with this basic circular movement for each arm, practise
them together.

1. *Hold your left hand up beside
your head, your palm turned to
face outward, your fingers slightly
spread. Your right hand is level
with your waist, its palm facing
your belly.*

2. *Move your left hand
away from your face in a
gentle arc. Gently turn your
palm outward. Your palm
leads the downward
movement.*

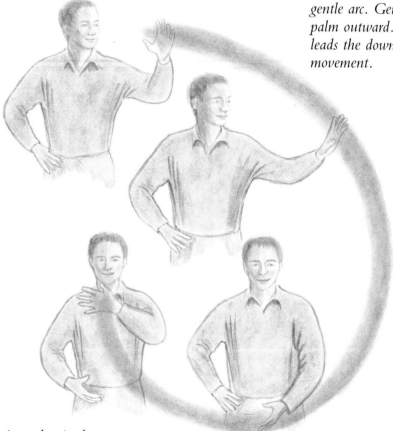

4. *Continue the circular movement
bringing your hand up in front of
your face ready to begin again.*

3. *At the bottom of the arc, your
hand starts to come up again.
Your palm faces your body.*

When you are comfortable with the arm movements of Waving Hands like Clouds, you can gently coordinate the motion of your hands, head and eyes.

1. *Imagine that your hands are floating through the atmosphere like clouds in the sky. Lazily you watch the clouds as they pass slowly by. To practise, begin with watching the movement of one hand. Turn your head so your gaze can follow the movement of the hand away from your body.*

2. *When your palm is turned away and moving outward from your head, start to bring your other hand up to begin its circle.*

3. *Calmly turn your head back towards the centre so you can see the palm of the other hand as it starts to move upward. Let your head and gaze naturally follow the palm with a soft focus.*

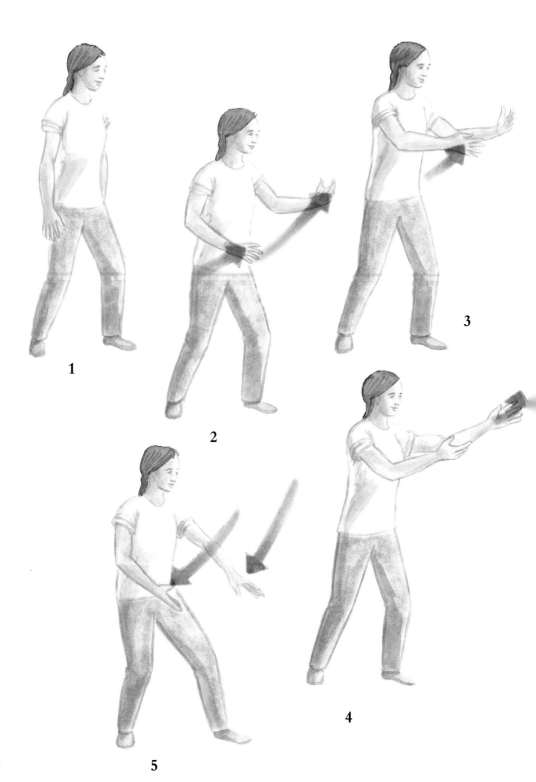

1

2

3

4

5

Reaching Outward and Pulling Back

This is one of the most classical movements found in the best known forms of Tai Chi. It helps to coordinate movement of the entire body, releasing tension in all the major joints of the body. It is part of a sequence often known as Grasping the Sparrow's Tail.

It should be performed like the graceful motion of a streamer in the breeze. The body sways slightly forward and backward with the hands moving effortlessly along with the movement.

1. Stand with your feet shoulder-width apart. Turn your hips toward the left and place your left foot so that it points toward the left. The angle between your right heel and left heel is 90 degrees. Shift 60 per cent of your weight on to your left foot.

2. Raise your left arm so that your left palm faces the centre of your chest. Imagine you are holding a large balloon between your forearm and your chest. Bring your right hand up near your hip.

3. Slowly sweep your right hand up. It stops, palm upward, as if you were supporting the imaginary balloon between your two palms.

4. Slowly move your left hand up and away from you as if you were reaching up to catch something in the air just ahead of you, level with your head.

5. Bring your weight back on to the right foot. Your right knee bends slightly as the weight transfers to that side. Bring your hands toward you at the same time as if you were carefully pulling a large object down toward your belly. Keep the same distance between your hands as they move.

Then continue the sequence by raising your left arm, as in figure 2, so that you make the movements into a smooth, continuous loop.

棚
攮

*Making the continuous
loop to the right side*

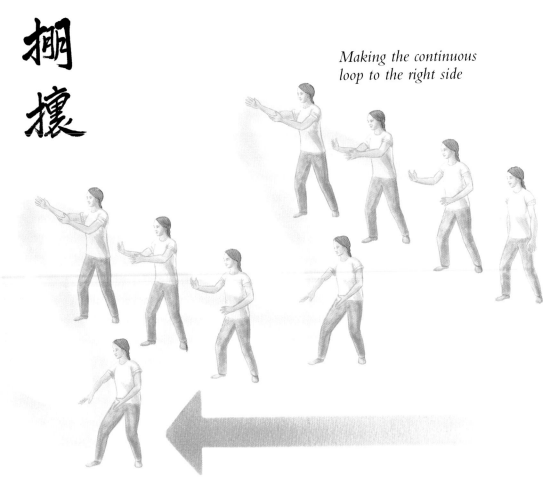

When you become familiar with the individual movements of Reaching Outward and Pulling Back, let them
flow freely and smoothly one after another. As you shift
your body weight forward and backward, begin with 60
per cent on your front foot and then shift to 60 per cent
on your rear foot. There should be no point at which
you stop. You are like a river whose energy is forever
flowing.

*Making the continuous
loop to the left side*

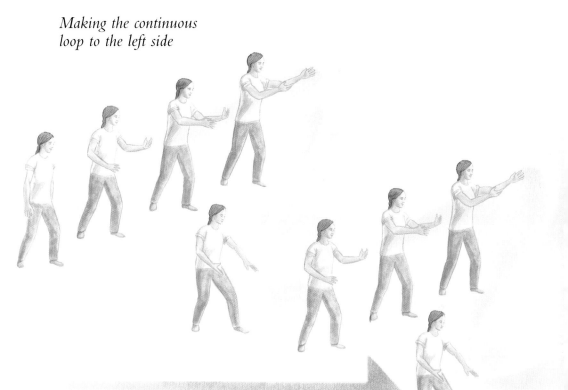

To ensure the smooth flow of Chi as you perform this flowing movement, try to avoid straightening or locking either your elbows or knees. Your arms and legs should always have a feeling of being relaxed. As you develop this feeling of slow, relaxed movement, make sure that your wrists and fingers move gracefully, as if they were the ends of long streamers in the air.

Begin by learning the basic movements. Then, when you are able to link them together, try performing the whole sequence 10 times to the left side. Stop, and turn to the right. Then perform the sequence 10 times to the right side. As you develop greater strength, work up to 30 sequences on each side.

Pressing Forward and Pushing Out

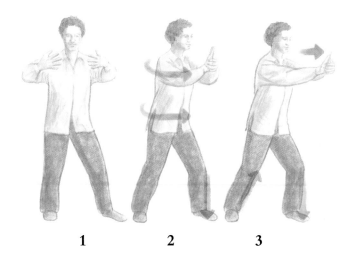

1   2   3

1. Start facing forward with your feet shoulder-width apart. Turn your left foot so that it points approximately 90 degrees to the left. Raise both your arms in front of you, as if you were holding a large balloon between your palms and your chest.

2. Turn your hips towards the left and shift your weight so that 60 per cent is on the left foot. Bring the heels of your hands together in a crossed position, looking like a butterfly with its wings spread. Both arms should be slightly bent at the elbows. Your left hand is outermost.

3. Slowly press forward using the power in your back leg to shift forward so that 70 per cent of your weight is on your left foot. Imagine that the ball between your arms and chest expands so that your arms move slightly outward. Keep your elbows bent.

This movement, also from Grasping the Sparrow's Tail, moves the body's energy more powerfully.

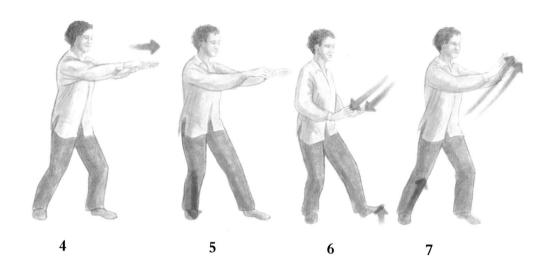

4   **5**   **6**   **7**

4. Separate your hands and turn both palms down. Move your hands away from each other in a horizontal line until they are shoulder-width apart. Your fingers face forward.

5. Your hands remain still. Carefully shift your weight back on to your right foot until 70 per cent is on your rear foot. Bend your right knee as you do this. Your torso remains upright, but your whole body feels that it is sinking down over the right foot.

6. At the same time, bring both your hands back and down in a diagonal movement toward your waist. Raise your left foot so that only the heel remains on the ground.

7. Using your right foot, steadily push yourself up and forward until 70 per cent of your weight is on the front foot. Extend your arms so that they move forward and upward. You finish with your torso upright. Your hands point gently upward at a 45-degree angle, level with your shoulders with your elbows gently bent.

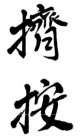

Once you have learned the individual movements, run the whole sequence together. You move like a wave in the ocean, your whole body expressing the increase of energy, its release and return. As you become more familiar with the sequence, you will feel your body moving as one unit, powered by the subtle shifts of weight between your feet.

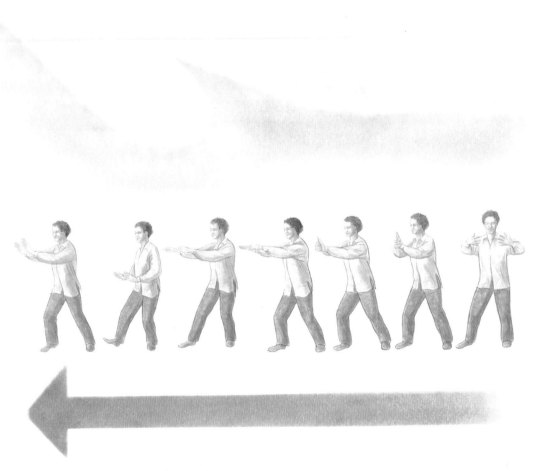

Making the continuous loop to the right side

Start by learning the correct
movements in the sequence.
Then aim to perform the
whole motion 10 times to
one side and then 10 times
to the other. When you feel
ready, build up to 30 on
each side.

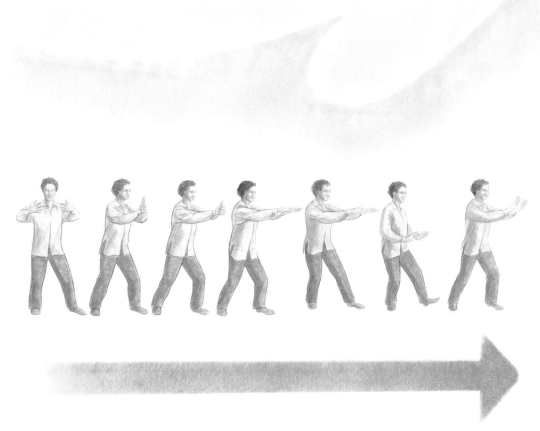

*Making the continuous
loop to the left side*

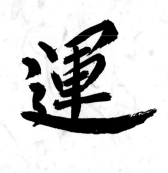

PART THREE

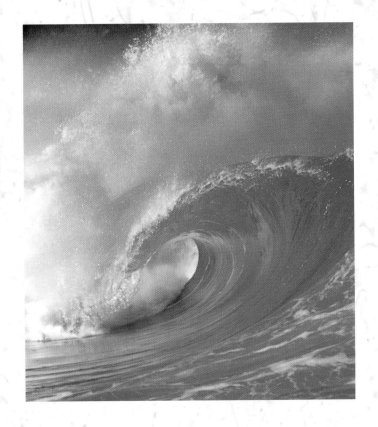

RIDING
THE
WAVES
Working with Inner Strength

Introduction

*Your internal organs are peaceful and your thoughts
are calm; your muscles are strong, your eyes and ears
are alert and clear. You have accurate perceptions and
understanding; you are firm and strong without
snapping.*

HUAI-NAN TZU

As you start to unlock the years of accumulated tension
in your body, your Chi naturally begins to increase and
flow more smoothly. Everyone experiences this change
differently. Much depends on the way in which the
stress has been locked into the body over the years.

The underlying transformation occurs in your
fundamental energy pattern. Your Chi is more stable.
Its flow becomes more even. You begin to feel that
something has become stronger within you. This
sensation of riding the waves corresponds to the energy
patterns described on pages 12 and 13:

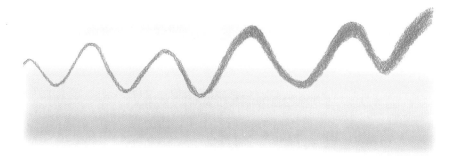

In this part of the book you are introduced to the
more powerful Zhan Zhuang positions. Practising
these will greatly increase the volume and flow of
your Chi. However, they are also more challenging
because they work on more deep-seated obstacles to
this higher potential.

You experience these challenges in two main ways. First, you may find that you go through a lot of muscular pain as you hold the positions. These pains are caused by excessive tension in your muscles. The antidote is to consciously relax the muscle fibres in the area where you feel the pain. The second challenge occurs in your nervous system. You may feel overwhelmed by great impatience, unbearable boredom, intense irritation. The sensations are the residue of years of stress. The antidote is to practise Calming the Spirit (see pages 38–9) as you stand.

There is one further point that is vital for all practitioners, regardless of their level of training. It applies to all the practices in this book, but it is all the more important when you start to hold the more demanding Zhan Zhuang positions to which you are introduced in this part of the book. Sometimes, practitioners may unconsciously end up looking rather grim. Their lips tighten and their eyes narrow. They look like they are taking sour medicine.

Remember that these are healing practices, not punishments. This understanding should be reflected in a soft smile. First let your face and neck muscles relax. You can briefly close your eyes as you do this. Then let a smile naturally form from within and express itself outwards as you open your eyes. Let your smile be your companion as you stand.

Practising regularly like this makes a great difference. It is far better to do five minutes day after day, and slowly build up the length of time, than to spend one day doing excessive practice as compensation for a week lost doing nothing!

直
胸
撑
拔

Holding the Balloon

Once you have learned to stand in Wu Chi (pages 34–5) for up to 10 minutes and are able to do this without too much difficulty, you can begin to practise this next position, Holding the Balloon.

This position is more strenuous and takes time to perfect. The effort involved greatly increases the flow of Chi in your system. This increased energy activity sometimes creates unusual sensations. Some people feel the strain in their muscles. Others experience tingling, like pins and needles. You may feel that your body has shifted out of its normal alignment. If your customary posture is slightly crooked or lop-sided, your inner balancing mechanism will be used to that. Therefore, when you are standing in the properly balanced and symmetrical Chi Kung position, it may take time for your nervous system and muscles to get used to this new feeling.

Begin by standing in Wu Chi. Your feet should be shoulder-width apart. To move into the new position, slowly sink down roughly 5 cm (2 in). Imagine that there is a stool behind you and that you are lowering yourself slightly to rest upon it. This will help you remain upright. Keep your weight evenly spread over the soles of your feet. Do not let your knees bend forwards over your toes.

Then slowly raise both your arms as if you were starting to embrace someone very gently in front of you. Bring your hands up level with your chest, but not as high as your shoulders. Your elbows should be slightly lower than your wrists.

The distance between the finger tips of your two hands should be approximately equivalent to the width of one of your fists.

Open your fingers so that there is space between each of them. Your thumbs should be slightly raised, but not tensed.

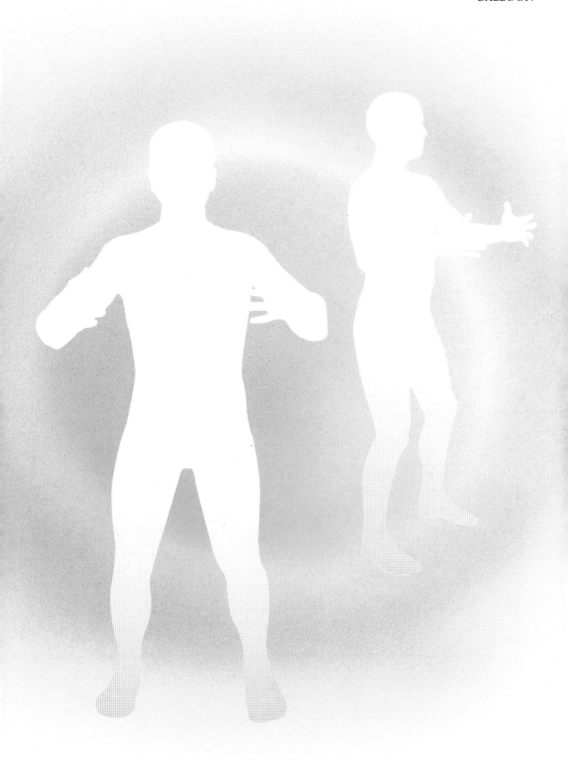

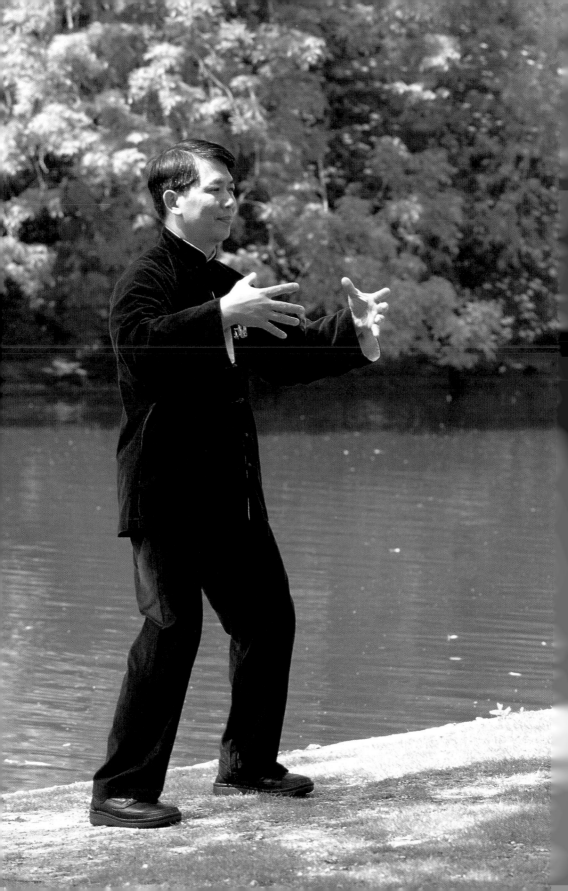

直
胸
撐
拔

When you have moved into the position for Holding the Balloon, you can then pay careful attention to the precise way in which you are standing. These details are important because the position, if held in the proper way, will start to correct subtle problems that you may have in your posture and clear hidden blockages in your internal energy pathways.

Feel as if you are holding a large, imaginary balloon between your open hands and your chest. Your hands are slightly curved around the inflated skin of the balloon. Be aware of the spaciousness between your arms and your chest, and also under your elbows and armpits.

Sometimes you may find that you have unconsciously raised your shoulders when moving your arms into the position. Let them relax and sink down.

Relax your chest. You can do this by releasing the muscle tension in your torso when you breathe out.

Pay attention to the way you are holding your head and neck. Your head should be upright, neither nodding forward nor angled backward or upward. Imagine the centre point of a line running across your skull between the tips of your ears. Feel that you are being gently suspended from that very point.

Make sure your chin is not protruding forward. It should be comfortably tucked in.

Your breathing should be completely natural. Do not try to adjust it in any way.

The inner work of this exercise is simply to stand still in this position for several minutes at a time. Begin with a couple of minutes, if you can manage that. Then increase, day by day, until you are able to stand for between 5 and 15 minutes, relaxed and motionless.

直胸撐拔

Relaxation in the Chi Kung positions is one of the secrets that will give you the maximum benefit from the practice. The method of relaxation is unique. Chi Kung relaxation is not like falling asleep or slumping down in a chair or numbing the mind. You remain alert, but you

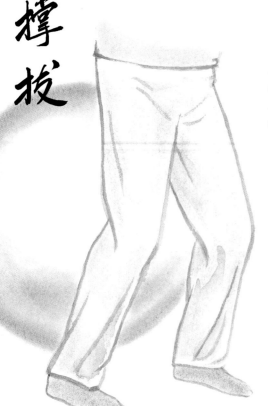

1. *The weight of your upper body is supported by a large imaginary balloon on which you feel you are sitting. Your spine sinks downward, your buttock muscles relax.*

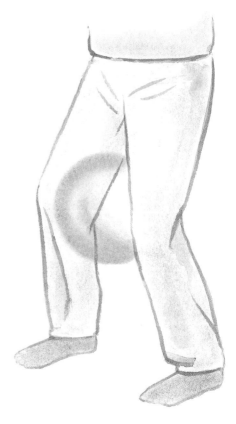

2. *There is a small imaginary balloon between your knees. You are applying just enough pressure to hold it in place, but you are not tense. This makes sure that you are using the muscles on the inner margin of your thighs and not letting your legs bow outward.*

are not stressed. The method is to focus your thoughts and feelings on the balloons shown below. As you become more familiar with this type of inner work, you will begin to feel completely supported as you stand and your relaxation will deepen.

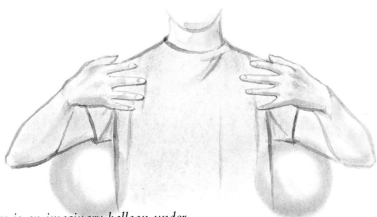

3. *There is an imaginary balloon under each of your armpits. This supports your upper arm. It keeps your arms away from your chest, allowing your lungs more freedom as you breathe. As you relax into the balloon, you feel the accumulated tension in your shoulders being released.*

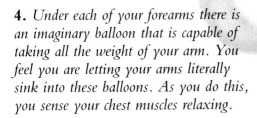

4. *Under each of your forearms there is an imaginary balloon that is capable of taking all the weight of your arm. You feel you are letting your arms literally sink into these balloons. As you do this, you sense your chest muscles relaxing.*

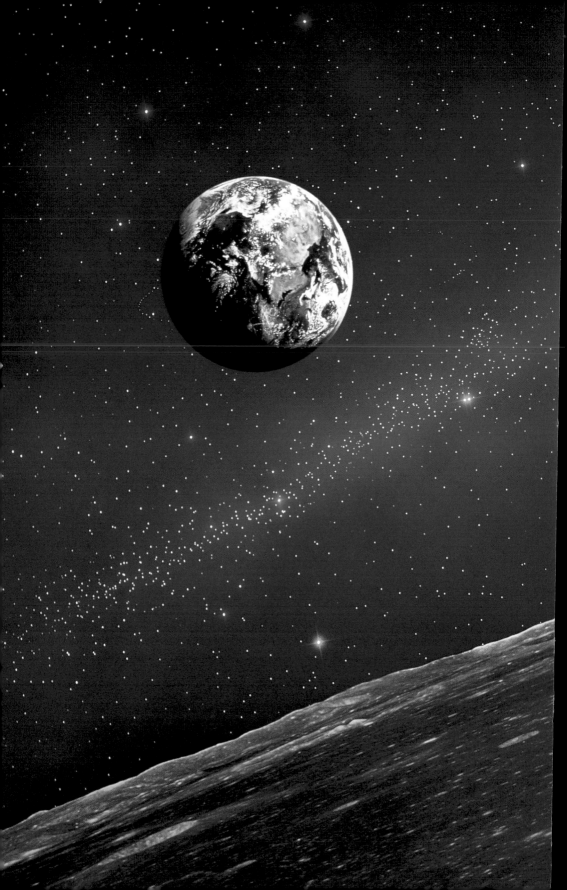

The Galaxy

The ancient Chinese philosopher Chuang-tse was famed for his profound love of nature. He felt a deep affinity with the entire cosmos. "Heaven, earth and I are living together, and all things and I form an inseparable unity," he wrote.

Sometimes when we look up into the sky at night and see the stars, we ask ourselves what it would be like to travel in space. It is as if we had forgotten everything that we have learned from the astronomers. The truth is that we *are* space travellers, hurtling through the cosmos with breathtaking speed.

In order to catch the signals from outer space we erect great circular dishes that attract and funnel the incoming energy into electronic receptors. We use the same principle for home satellite television reception.

In our own very personal way, we are doing the same thing when we practise Chi Kung. Each of us is a sensitive reception point for the energy that surrounds us. We are travelling through the galaxy, influenced by its signals and attracting its power. This process takes place naturally all the time, and our capacity to draw on that power is dramatically enhanced by the practice of Chi Kung.

When we stand in the position known as Holding the Balloon, the circle of our arms literally acts as a reception dish. It is as if we had opened up an unfolding antenna to the universe. The more we relax into that position and the longer we practise, the more sensitive we become to the energy that flows around us and through us.

As our practice develops, we begin to understand through our own direct experience, the intimate meaning of Chuang-tse: "Heaven, earth and I are living together."

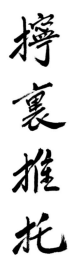

Opening Outward

This next Chi Kung position takes your personal development to a new threshold. It should be practised only after you are comfortable with the previous position, Holding the Balloon, and have been able to build up regular practice of at least 15 minutes a day.

This new position helps to develop your stamina. It makes greater demands on the muscles in your legs and arms. It also makes greater demands on your nervous system: you are tempted to give up and it requires increased patience to hold this position without moving.

If you are just starting to learn this position, you should be careful to begin with a warm-up. First, do one or two of the movement exercises in Part Two that you like best. Then stand in Wu Chi for five minutes, followed by Holding the Balloon for a further five minutes.

You have already lowered yourself by about 5 cm (2 in) when moving into Holding the Balloon. Now you go lower, being careful not to let your knees bend forward over your toes. Try to keep your body upright as you do this to prevent pushing your bottom outward.

As you go lower, you feel the pull on your thigh muscles. This increased effort immediately starts to step up your blood circulation, demonstrating the old Chi Kung saying: "The legs are the second heart".

Despite the increased effort involved, remind yourself to relax. Try to release the tension in your lower back and buttocks.

Then raise your arms and turn your palms outward, away from your face, so that the backs of your hands are level with your eyes.

Your fingers remain slightly spread with your palms and thumbs relaxed.

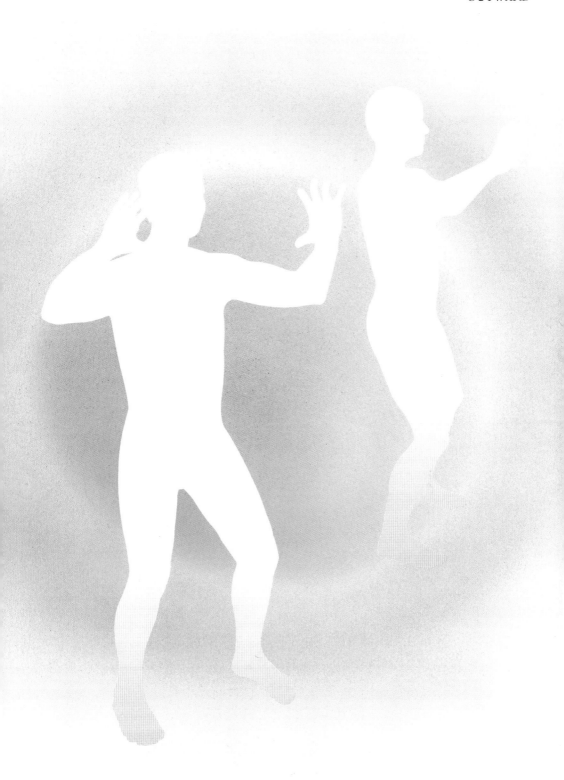

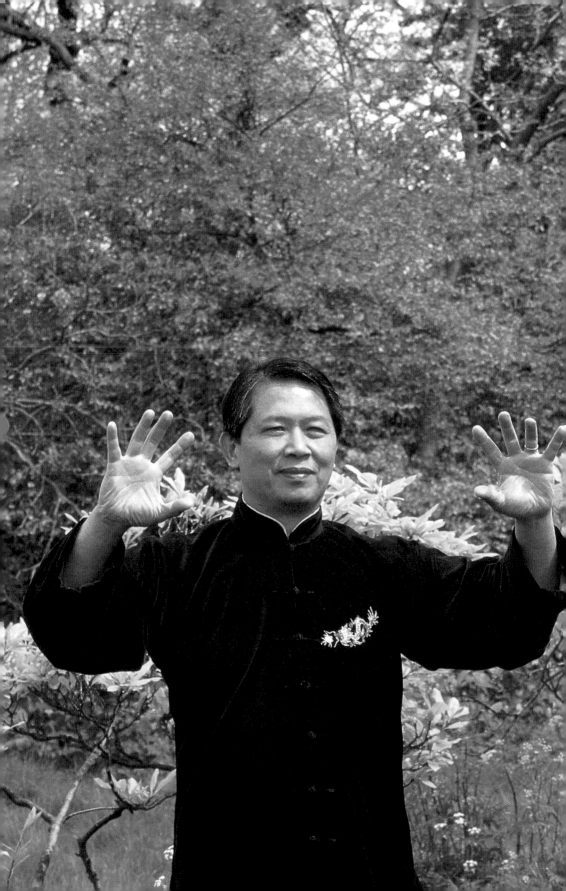

擰
裹
推
托

When you adopt this position, you feel a strong surge of
Chi. You may feel an increase in body heat and begin
to sweat. You may feel intensified tingling in the fingers
or skin. This is sometimes called "the echo of the Chi".
You may have shaking or trembling sensations. These
are caused by the rush of Chi encountering obstacles in
the energy pathways and beating against them like
waves.

You should start holding this position for short periods
of time. It is more important to work on getting the
position correct, even if only briefly, rather than strug-
gling for a long time in a distorted posture. For some
people, it will be more than enough to hold the position correctly for half a minute to begin with. Build up
gradually, always remembering the importance of
relaxing into the position.

If you find that it is extremely difficult to hold the position, you can rise up slightly so that you are not sinking
down quite as low. That will ease the pain in your legs.
You can gently lower your arms back to Holding the
Balloon. That will relieve pain in your arms. You can
scan your body, making an effort to relax the muscles
and flesh wherever you pinpoint tension.

Just as in Holding the Balloon (see pages 82–3), you
imagine you are sitting on a large balloon and holding
one between your knees. Other balloons support your
upper arms. Imagine all of these bearing your weight.

To hold this position correctly, be aware of spaciousness
and lightness surrounding your arms and hands. Feel the
space in front of your open hands, as if you were resting
your palms on an invisible support in front of you.

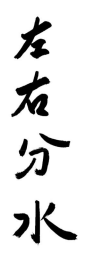

Extending to the Sides

As your energy develops through Chi Kung practice, it begins to act like a powerful current flowing with greater and greater strength from deep inside you right out to the furthest margins of your body. This next position, Extending to the Sides, encourages this process. It also helps you remain stable while experiencing the increased flow of Chi.

Start to practise this position after you have developed some experience of Opening Outward, where you should be able to hold your hands up at the level of your head for at least 3–5 minutes.

Begin in Wu Chi and hold it for 5 minutes. Then move into Holding the Balloon, and remain in this position for a further 5 minutes.

Sink a little lower, going down an additional 5 cm (2 in). Make sure that your knees do not protrude forward over your toes. You should feel that your entire upper body weight is resting on the imaginary large balloon under your buttocks. This sense of sinking downward is extremely important as it develops your ability to connect with the energy of the Earth.

Slowly move both your arms down and out toward the sides. Your hands should be level with your waist, slightly in front of you. Your hands are relaxed, with your fingers gently spread apart.

Be careful not to hunch your shoulders or to lock your elbows or wrists.

If you are already capable of standing in the previous position, Opening Outward, for at least 3–5 minutes without moving, you will likely find that you can maintain this position for 5 minutes. Aim for that if you can, and then increase the length of time until you are able to stand motionless in this position for 10 minutes.

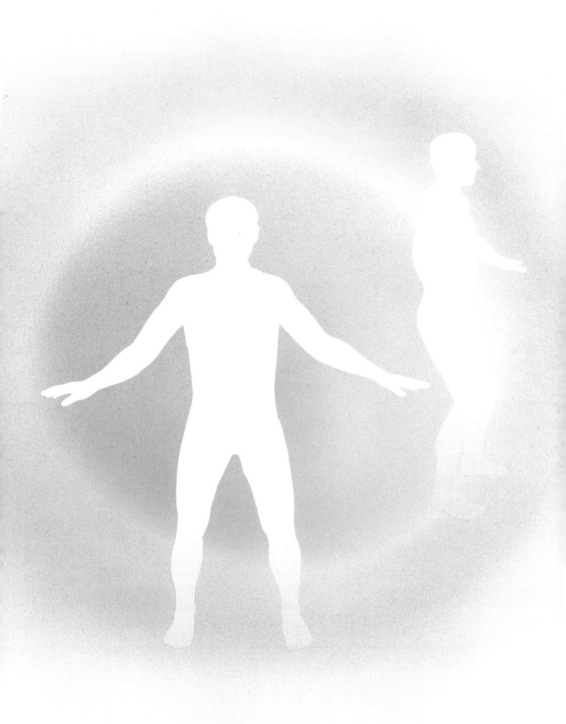

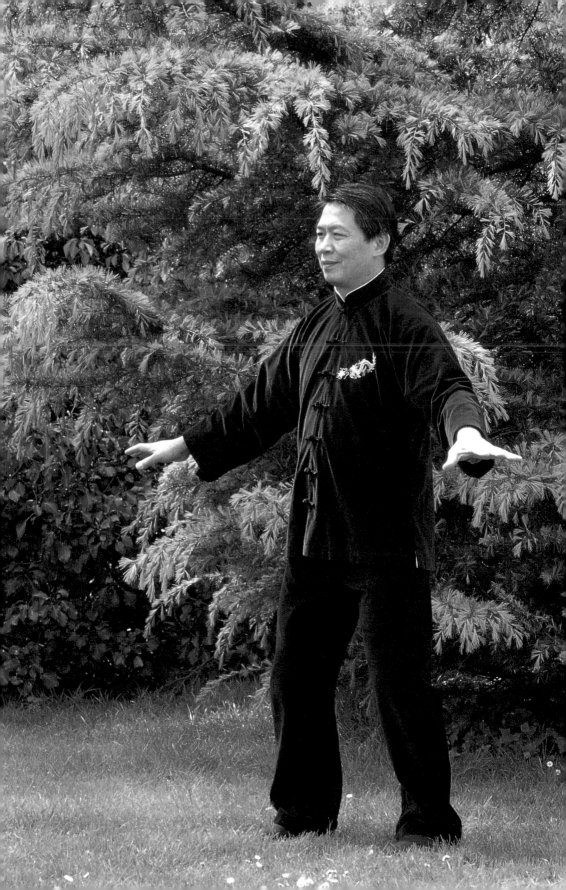

左
右
分
水

When you see great masters practising Chi Kung it is
hard at first to imagine what is going on. It is clear that
they are engaged in some form of activity, but at the
same time there is also sense of quiescence, as if they are
inwardly experiencing profound tranquillity.

To achieve this, your mind needs to be fully engaged in
the practice. In this position, Extending to the Sides,
you again call to mind a number of imaginary balloons
which are essential to the inner relaxation.

First, there is the large imaginary balloon on which you
are resting your buttocks. Focus your attention on the
balloon, so that you are able to relax your back fully.
You should have the feeling that you are sinking as
much of your weight into the balloon as possible.

Then there is the little imaginary balloon between your
knees. Just try to keep it gently in place, so you maintain the subtle alignment of your legs.

As in the previous positions, there are also the two
imaginary balloons under your armpits, keeping your
upper arms gently supported away from your torso.

There are four other balloons that you visualize while
holding this position. Two of them are under your
hands. It is as if these balloons were floating in a stream
of water. The water gives them additional buoyancy, so
that they can take all the weight of your outstretched
arms. The current in the stream also gives these balloons
a vitality so that you feel them constantly moving under
your palms. The stream would carry them away if you
were not keeping them ever so gently under your
control.

The other two balloons are resting on top the backs of
your outstretched hands. Like an accomplished juggler,
you are keeping them effortlessly poised in position.

The Full Sequence

When you have learned the basic standing positions you can put them together in a complete sequence. Your entire energy system will be refreshed and your nervous system calmed. Take time to go through the sequence in the most relaxed manner possible.

Put on some soft instrumental music and close your eyes.

Make the transition between each position slowly and smoothly.

To begin with, and after each position, you gather your energy into your Tan Tien by standing with your hands held over your belly.

This is the position, Gathering your Chi, on pages 26–7.

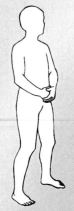

2 minutes

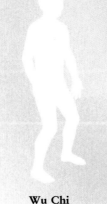

Wu Chi
3–5 minutes

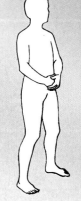

2 minutes

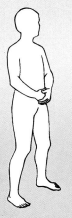

2 minutes

Extending to the Sides
3–5 minutes

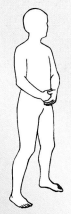

2 minutes

Opening Outward
3–5 minutes

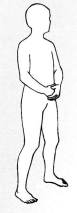

2 minutes

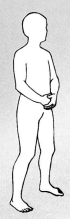

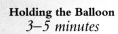

Holding the Balloon
3–5 minutes

2 minutes

The Full Belly
3–5 minutes

95

Strengthening the Golden Sphere

As your Chi grows in strength and volume it courses through your body with increasing power. This exercise, Strengthening the Golden Sphere, helps you become accustomed to an ever increasing flow of Chi. It also helps you to develop your hands as conduits for your Chi.

You can add this exercise after you have held any of the standing positions in this part of the book.

Stand with your feet shoulder-width apart, feet facing forward.

Bend your knees slightly, taking care not to lean forward over your toes.

Relax your backside, so that you feel a lengthening in the base of your spine and an easing of any tension in your upper body.

Imagine you are holding a golden sphere between your open palms, just in front of your abdomen. The sphere has the resilient quality of a fully inflated beach ball.

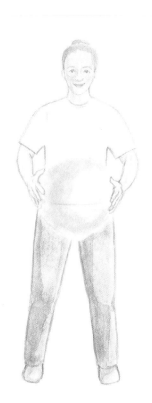

Practise making three separate
movements with your hands:
squeezing, shaking and turning.

1. *First, squeeze your palms together
as if you were trying to compress the
inflated ball, then immediately release
them back to their starting position.
Start slowly to get the feeling of
resilience between your palms, then
increase your speed.*

2. *Second, shake the ball up and
down between your hands as if
you were playing a shaker in the
rhythm section of a band. Imagine
the ball is heavy and try to shake
it fairly quickly.*

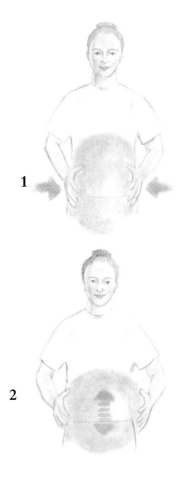

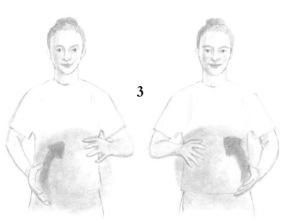

3. *Third, turn the ball over so that
your hands alternate being on top.
Try to do this as quickly as you can,
always keeping the feeling of the
sphere between your palms.*

Once you are able to make the three separate movements, try
to combine them randomly – sometimes pressing, suddenly
shaking, then turning, turning and pressing at the same time
and so on.

Practise for about five minutes. Then fold your hands over your
abdomen to conclude with Gathering your Chi (see pages 26–7).

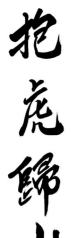

The Tiger and the Mountain

This is the final, powerful movement of most classical
Tai Chi forms. It is usually known by its full name:
Embracing the Tiger and Returning to the Mountain.
This poetic expression conveys the two essential
qualities of the movement. The Tiger symbolizes the
full power which is generated by the practice. This is a
force that the practitioner gradually comes to embrace,
enjoy and completely express. The Mountain is the
inner stillness that is said to be "the mother of motion".
Your power emerges out of that stillness and it is to that
same stillness that you return.

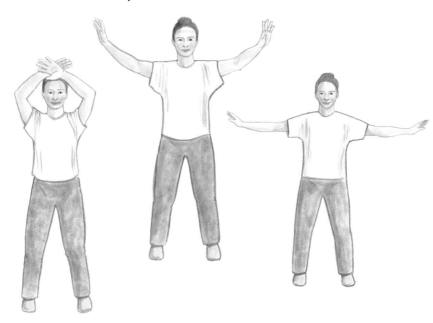

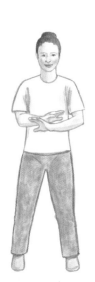

The specific elements of the movement are described in
detail on pages 100–3. The whole sequence is shown
here so that you can clearly see how the entire
movement sweeps along. You begin in stillness. Then
your arms open wide and you go down as if to lift the
Tiger up in your arms. You rise up with the Tiger in
your embrace. Then, as you straigthen up and turn
your palms downward, you are still – returning to
the Mountain.

Coordinating your breathing

*It is important to coordinate your breathing with
the main phases of this movement. First stand
still, breathing naturally. As you start the
movement, breathe in as you raise your arms. As
your arms start to circle downward, breathe out.
When you reach the lowest position and begin to
come up, breathe in. As you turn your palms
down at the end and complete rising up, breathe
out. If you feel tired, stand still breathing
naturally before starting the movement again.*

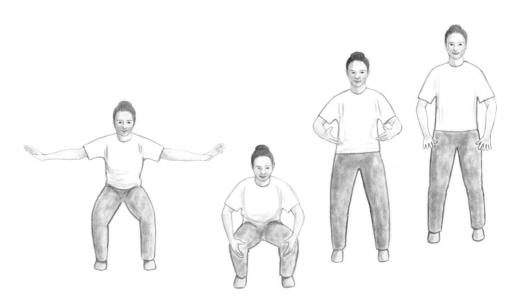

Calmly and slowly complete 10 full
movements. Later you can advance to 30
or more.

To finish, let your hands slowly come to rest
by your sides. Stand still for a minute,
allowing your internal energies to balance
and flow smoothly.

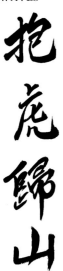

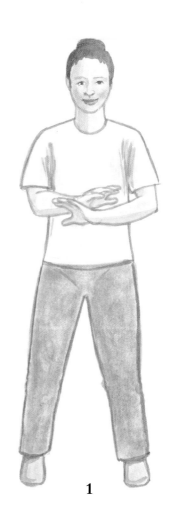

1. *Stand with your feet facing forward, shoulder-width apart. Your knees are slightly bent. Cross your arms in front of you with both your palms facing away from you. The front of your right wrist is against the back of your left wrist. Breathe naturally.*

1

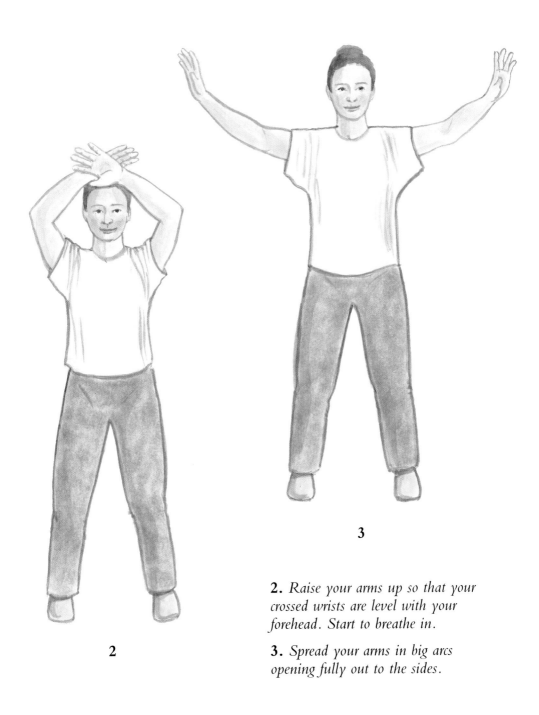

3

2

2. *Raise your arms up so that your crossed wrists are level with your forehead. Start to breathe in.*

3. *Spread your arms in big arcs opening fully out to the sides.*

抱
虎
歸
山

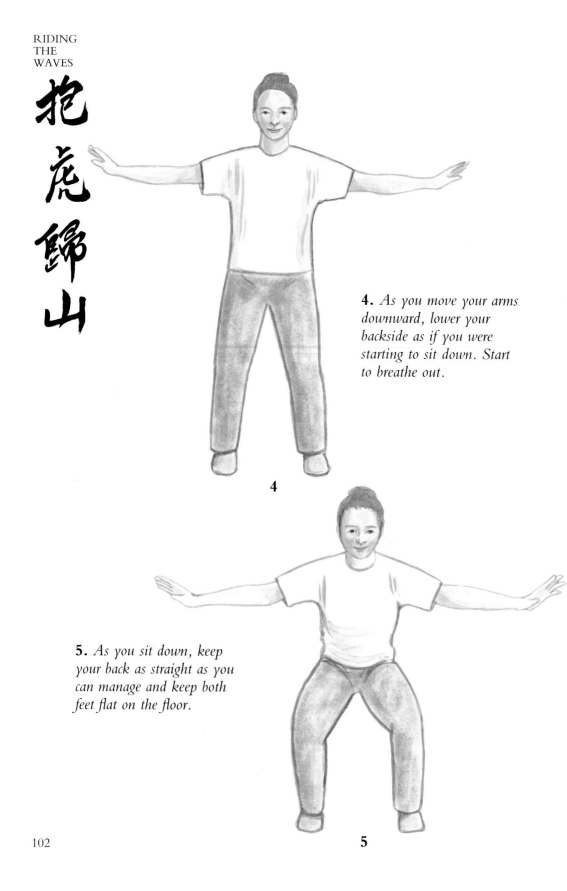

4. *As you move your arms downward, lower your backside as if you were starting to sit down. Start to breathe out.*

4

5. *As you sit down, keep your back as straight as you can manage and keep both feet flat on the floor.*

5

8. *Turn both your hands over so that the palms face downward. Breathe out. You finish standing up, but ending with your knees slightly bent, as at the beginning. You are ready to repeat the movement.*

7. *Lift both your hands up in front of you as if you were lifting a large basin, until they are level with your chest. Start to stand up at the same time that you lift your hands. Breathe in.*

6. *When you have gone as low as you can, bring both arms down so that your hands are opposite your abdomen.*

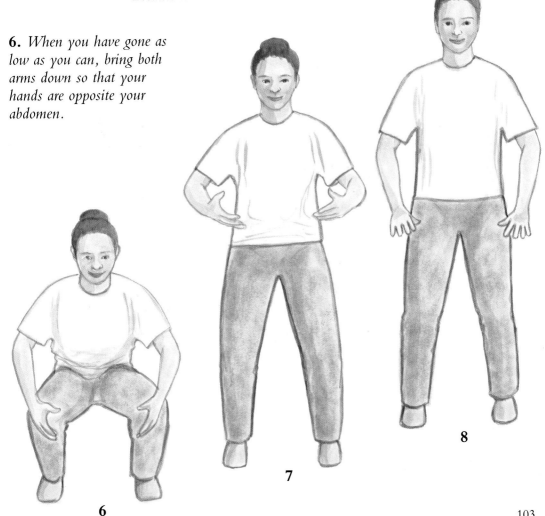

6

7

8

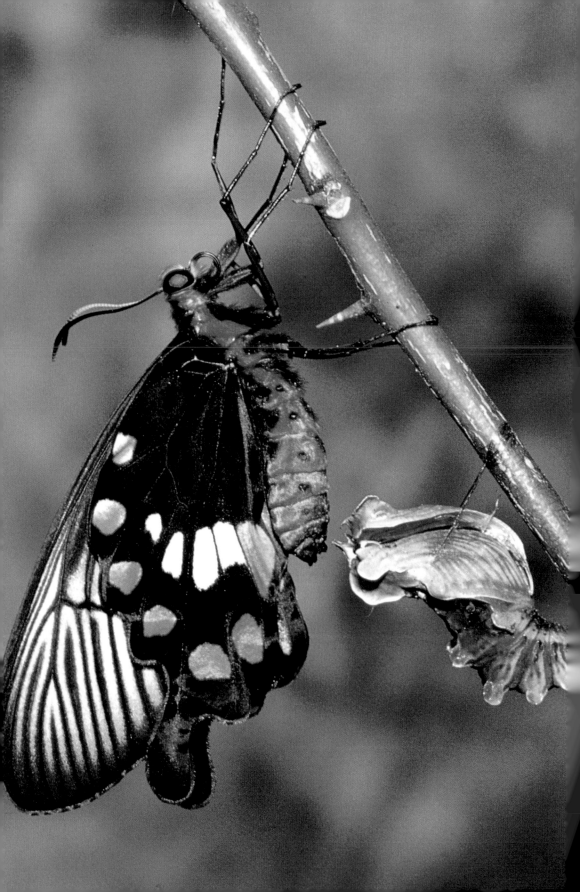

The Butterfly

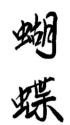

Although each of us is a part of nature, we often fail to understand its workings. We are often oblivious even to the changes in our own bodies.

When we practise Chi Kung we change. When we stand in the postures of Zhan Zhuang, those changes begin in profound and subtle ways. They affect virtually every aspect of our being – right down to the circulation of our blood cells and the functioning of our nerves.

These changes begin within and are unseen. They take time and careful work – as the masters say, like the way a butterfly emerges from the caterpillar's form.

The butterfly begins its work in stillness. Out of its own body, it spins its chrysalis. It draws its power inward to itself, ceases all movement, and begins its journey to new life.

The chrysalis itself is motionless. From time to time it sways a little in the breeze. It is easily mistaken for an autumn leaf.

Within the chrysalis, life's pattern starts to change. The work is silent and invisible. Until one day, the energy – renewed, repatterned and refreshed – emerges in the light.

Like every birth, it seems miraculous. Like a blossom opening from its bud, like a child's eyes opening after sleep, we find ourselves in the presence of nature's great transforming power.

Before, the butterfly was earthbound, first sealed inside its crawling body, then its chrysalis. Now, poised for flight, its mind takes wing.

行為活迎

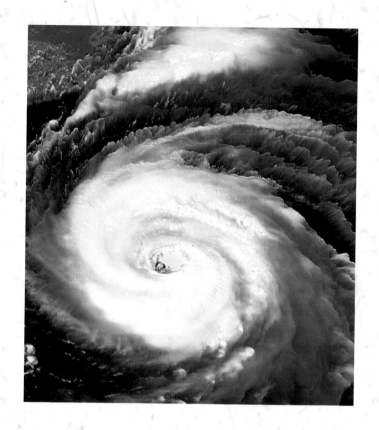

PART FOUR

REMOVING
THE
OBSTACLES
Healing yourself and Others

Introduction

*The three treasures of vitality, energy and spirit
experience a daily flourishing of life and fill the whole
body, so that the great medicine can be expected to be
produced naturally.*

CHUANG-TSE

It takes time and patience to mature in the practice of
Chi Kung. The transformation takes place slowly, like a
gradual change in your metabolic rate. Because the
practice is so personal, it is not easy to predict in
advance the changes that will occur in each person.

As you make progress, however, both the quality and
quantity of your Chi will change. Your Chi will
become more and more like a broad river. It will be
strong and smooth flowing. It will be available to you
like a well filled with fresh water. You will feel as if you
are riding on the back of an invisible, powerful creature.
This is the pattern of high energy, "Radiating
Outward", described on page 13.

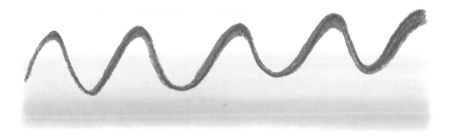

This high level of energy gives you increased stamina,
more emotional resilience and the ability to face difficulties with greater confidence. You start to recover
more rapidly from injuries and illnesses.

Your mental alertness will be sharper. Your sense of humour may be heightened, as will your visual and other sensory acuity. In tests conducted in China, people who practised Zhan Zhuang were found to respond to random signals five times faster than others.

This increased energy acts like a powerful magnetic field. Its power can be used for self-healing and to help others. In this part of the book you are shown how to use your hands as healing instruments. You are introduced to a system of massage based on the classical Chinese Theory of the Five Energies and shown how this system can be used, together with the results of your Chi Kung practice, to help overcome the obstacles to a balanced flow of energy in the body.

This massage technique results from the merging of three systems: the Zhan Zhuang tradition of Chi Kung as taught by Great Grand Master Wang Xiang Zhai in China in the earlier part of this century; orthodox Western medicine practised by Professor Yu Yong Nian, a former student of Great Grand Master Wang and the authority responsible for introducing Chi Kung therapy into hospitals in China; and the Traditional Chinese Medicine studied and practised by the author, who introduced Zhan Zhuang to the West.

This massage system will only work for practitioners who have reached a reasonably advanced level of Zhan Zhuang practice. If you have carefully followed the instructions in the earlier part of this book, you will likely find that you can use this system to heal localised injuries and pain that you experience yourself. Later, as you gain experience, you will find you are able to use your powerful Chi to help your friends and family.

Hands of Bliss

During the Tang dynasty, Master Pai Chang instructed his students by using the example of a little boy who goes out to herd oxen. At first the young oxherd cannot even find an ox.

After searching he catches glimpses of one, and then eventually learns how to tame it and ride it. Over the centuries, beautiful brush paintings have been used to depict the progress of the little oxherd. Known as The Ten Oxherding Pictures, they have inspired generations of practitioners. The tenth picture, Entering the Marketplace with Bliss Bestowing Hands, is startling because it seems to have nothing to do with oxherding. Instead, it depicts a portly figure carrying a sack. The old man is said to be the monk, Pu Tai, often thought to be the origin of the figure we know today as The Laughing Buddha.

His great belly symbolizes his immense Chi and his huge sack is filled with whatever is needed to benefit others:

"Bare-chested and bare-footed I enter the market – Without using magic, even the trees come to life before me."

The bliss bestowing hands of Chi Kung practitioners are literally the hands of people who, like the oxherd, have found and tamed their own energy. What began as a search for health becomes a process of self-healing. Having learned how to heal ourselves, we are then able to help others.

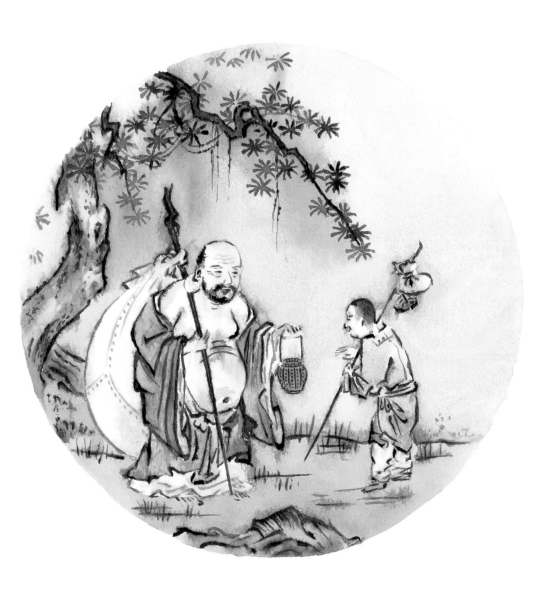

The Two Poles

As you develop your practice of Chi Kung, your hands act as increasingly powerful conduits of energy. They are like the terminals of an electric current. At any one time, one of these poles is positive, the other is negative. As your sensitivity increases and your Chi becomes more and more powerful, you can feel the invisible current running between your palms.

There are numerous healing applications of this current. Your two hands can be used in exactly the same way that magnets are used in magnet therapy. By placing your hands at different points on the body, the current passes through the body between your palms.

You can think of the person's body – or the part of the body that lies between your hands – as a small planet, like our own earth. The energy field between your hands is exactly like the energy of the galaxy that surrounds the earth and sustains its biosphere.

This healing application, The Two Poles, can be used as a form of first aid in many situations. For example, if a person has just stumbled and wrenched their ankle, you can apply your palms on either side of the affected area. This calms the nervous reaction, steadies the entire area and, depending on what has happened, can relieve the pain, swelling and internal haemorrhaging.

If you have not practised Zhan Zhuang Chi Kung regularly, have been practising incorrectly or have only been practising for a relatively short period of time, you should not expect to achieve miraculous results. But if you practise regularly and experience the sensations of the energy current between your palms, you can use your Chi in a number of applications, described over the following pages.

Preparing the current

Before performing the Chi Kung massage techniques
described over the following pages, you need to ensure
that there is a strong flow of Chi to your hands.

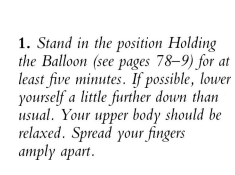

1. *Stand in the position Holding
the Balloon (see pages 78–9) for at
least five minutes. If possible, lower
yourself a little further down than
usual. Your upper body should be
relaxed. Spread your fingers
amply apart.*

2. *Clap your hands together about
a dozen times.*

3. *When you have completed
your standing, rub your palms
rapidly together for a few seconds
to warm them.*

You are now ready to work.

The Five Energies

There are five fundamental movements of energy. Forces move outward and inward, rise and descend, and rotate. The study of these movements forms the basis of one of the most famous systems in all Chinese wisdom, known as the Theory of the Five Energies.

The Chi Kung practitioner needs to know how to use the various forms of the Five Energies when treating any condition. Practical examples of these methods are given on pages 126–33.

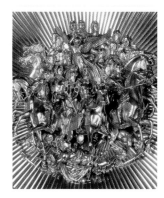

Metal

Metal is the most dense of all forms of matter. Its characteristic motion is the movement of energy inward. In the same way that metals are used to conduct electricity and to join materials together, Metal energy has a magnetic quality that pulls other energies toward it and binds forces together. In the Chinese calendar, Metal energy corresponds to the lunar phase of the waning moon. In the seasons, it is the Fall of the year, when nature draws in to itself.

Water

Water's energy descends. This is the state in which things reach their point of maximum rest and concentration. It is therefore the energy of regeneration. Water energy determines our fundamental constitution, giving us the power to exist, grow, act and reproduce. It is the basis of our willpower and motivation. It is like the new moon which, although dark, is about to emerge again into the light. It is the energy of Winter: still, hidden, awaiting rebirth.

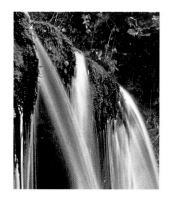

Wood

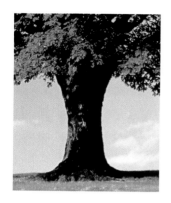

Wood symbolizes energy that expands outward like a tree. Like a tree in health, Wood energy keeps us strong, yet supple. It keeps us in balance with our environment and ensures the harmony of our inner functions. In the Chinese calendar, Wood energy corresponds to the waxing moon, as its energy increases and expands. This is the phase in the cycle at which things emerge and begin to grow. It is the energy which enables all of Nature to give birth. It is the energy of Spring.

Fire

Without Fire energy in the body, we would be cold and lifeless. Our inner fire sustains the multitude of chemical and biological processes. Fire is the radiating energy that gives rise to the emotional, mental and spiritual power of all the other organs. It is the spirit of life, giving us consciousness, the ability to appreciate life and the power to direct our lives. It connects us to the Universe and other beings. Fire is an emblem for human warmth, enabling us to communicate, share with others and be compassionate.

Earth

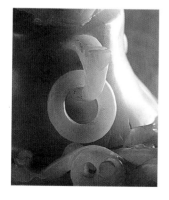

Earth energy moves horizontally. Its directions are lateral and circular, like the orbits of the planets. In the Chinese calendar, Earth energy is also understood to represent the period of change between each of the seasons. It is like the moon before it wanes – when it is closest to the earth – large, golden and full. Like the earth itself, it is patient, supportive and nurturing. It underpins, absorbs, withstands and accommodates all changes.

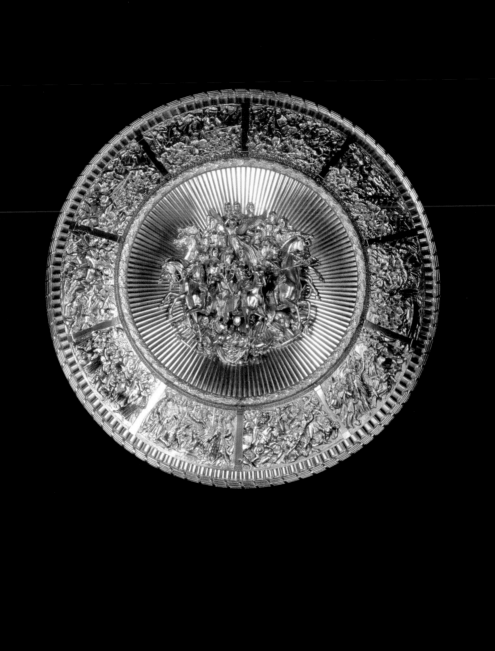

The Healing Energy of Metal

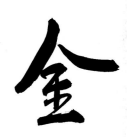

Some injuries and inner disturbances cause our Chi to disperse. Blood may drain away from the area, leaving it weak and cold. A Chi Kung practitioner can use the effect of their own Chi to restore the natural energy flow in the area which has been weakened. This can be done using Metal energy massage.

Metal energy moves inward. It is this inward, centripetal motion that creates the density and strength of all metallic substances in the natural world.

The precise method of Metal energy massage is to support the limb or other part of the body with one hand. Use the other hand to apply the massage technique. The idea is to use your hand to draw Chi in toward the affected area. You do this by making a series of strokes that move inward towards the centre of the area. It is as if you were tracing the lines of all the spokes of a chariot wheel as they run in from the rim of the wheel to the hub.

There are two styles of movement you can choose between, according to your preference and comfort.

One style is simply to make strokes that are single, straight and smooth. Use your whole palm and fingers for each stroke, if you can, in the space available. If you are working in a very narrow area, use the tips of a few fingers or your thumb.

The second style is to make each stroke like a series of tiny circles working inward along the line toward the centre of the area. You can make either clockwise or counter-clockwise circles, according to what is most comfortable for you.

If the person on whom you are working is very strong and they do not feel intense pain in the area, you can make these strokes with a fair degree of pressure. If the person is weak or cannot bear any pressure, make lighter movements on the surface of the skin.

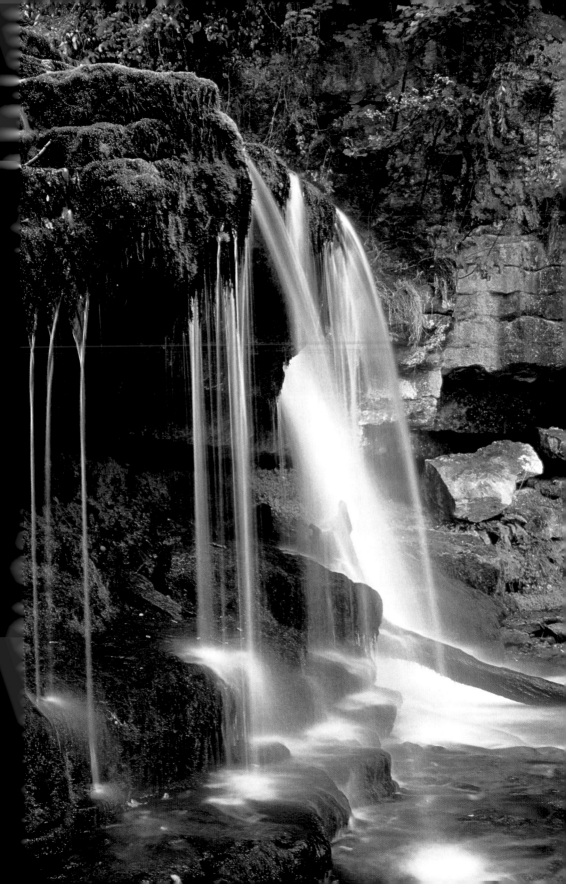

The Healing Energy of Water

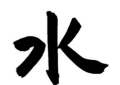

Water seeks the lowest level. It moves downward.

A Chi Kung practitioner can use Water energy massage to induce downward movements of Chi in areas where it has become congested. It can be used to help reduce swellings and relieve pains.

If you are working on a part of the body that you can hold in one hand then support it with one hand and use the other hand to make the massage movement. If you are working on the back or another area on which you can place both hands, place one hand near the affected area for support and control and use your other hand to perform the massage.

There are three styles of movement for Water energy massage. You can choose among them, depending on which feels best for you to work with. This may change from person to person and from time to time.

The first style is to create a vibration effect with your palm on and around the affected area. It is as if you were setting up a pattern of vibrations or ripples in a pond of water. You hold your palm firmly on the person's body and let your hand naturally shake or tremble, so that the vibrations go down into their underlying flesh, muscles and bones.

The second style is to create the same vibration effect, using your thumb only. This pressure is more focused, since the tip of the thumb covers such a small area. If the person does not find this too painful, work all around the affected area and, if possible, directly on it.

The third style is to press on or around the point, using your whole hand. If you are working on an area of the arms or legs, you can squeeze the affected area, using your fingers on one side of the limb to increase the pressure of your palm on the other side. The purpose of the massage remains the same: to allow your pressure to penetrate the area and descend as deeply as possible.

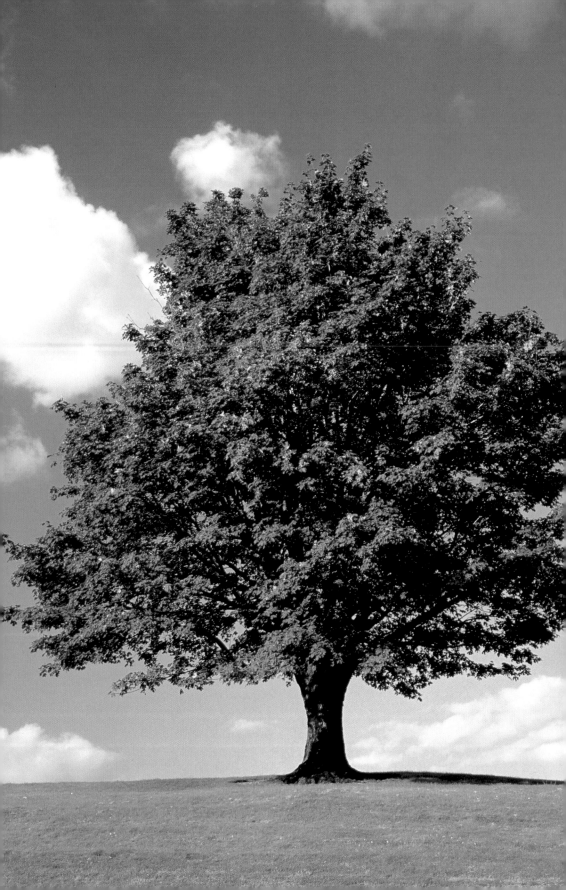

The Healing Energy of Wood

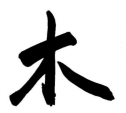

The normal tendency of Chi is to move. If there is an injury or sharp blow to the body, the Chi in the surrounding areas will instantly flow toward the site to provide support and protection. However, just as traffic can become congested as a result of a sudden increase in volume, the Chi can become blocked as it builds up.

The Chi Kung practitioner can help restore the normal flow of Chi by dispersing the blockage. The method for doing this is to use Wood energy massage. Just like the concentric rings in the heartwood of a tree, this energy moves outward from the centre – and can be used to draw other energy along with it.

The precise method of application is to use both hands. If you are working on a part of the body, such as a limb, that you can hold in one hand, then support it with one hand and use the other hand to do the massage movement. If you are working on the back or another area on which you can place both hands, place one hand near the affected area for support and control and use your other hand to perform the massage.

The purpose of this massage movement is to disperse any energy which has been blocked in the area. The movements radiate outwards from the affected area.

There are two styles of movement you can choose between. This is entirely a matter of personal preference. It may depend on the area on which you are working, your own inclination or the ease with which you are able to make the movements.

One style is to place your entire hand over the area and make a series of strokes which move outward from a central point. The pattern of movement resembles a primitive drawing of the many rays of the sun.

The second style is to make exactly the same pattern of movement using your thumb instead of your palm.

The Healing Energy of Fire

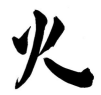

The potential of Fire energy is explosive. It moves upward, like a firework. But it is also penetrating.

Traditional Chinese doctors use heat to draw inner poisons from the body. Once, a section of hollow bamboo stem was sealed at one end and then stored in water. When needed, the inner core was heated up and the bamboo placed over the affected area. As the heat withdrew from the inside of the bamboo to the cool, outer surface, a hot vacuum was created that withdrew toxins from the body. The modern version of this is known as "cupping", using small heated glass bowls.

As you develop your internal power through the practice of Chi Kung, you will be able to accomplish similar results using the heat of your open palms. They are placed over the affected area, and then suddenly withdrawn, as if pulling adhesive from the skin. Like magnets, your hands extract energies blocked under the skin or deeper within the body.

This type of treatment has no harmful side effects. It is said to be like placing a stick into a hole in the ground to see if there is a snake inside. If a hidden poison emerges, it will rise naturally through the flesh, perhaps producing a pimple or some tenderness as it passes through the skin over the following days. The treatment itself causes no harm.

The precise method of application is to support the limb or other part of the body with one hand. Use the other hand to apply the massage technique. Hold that hand firmly over the affected area and penetrate the area by pressing down through your palm. Then abruptly and forcefully withdraw your hand upwards, as if unblocking a drain with a plunger.

Repeat the action several times.

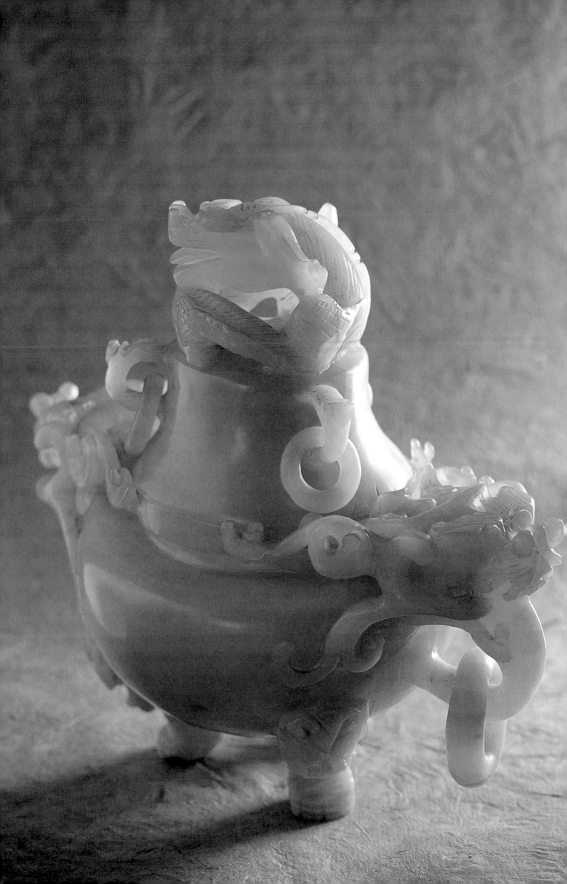

The Healing Energy of Earth

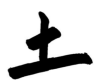

As the earth rotates around the sun, it describes an elipse, travelling in a constant plane. This calm, continuous motion is used in Earth energy massage. It relaxes the body and quiets the mind.

Earth energy massage is often used to open and close a Chi Kung massage treatment session. At the beginning, it is like a gentle warm-up. Then, like a relaxing cool-down at the end of an exercise, it provides the perfect completion to the treatment.

If you are working on a part of the body that you can hold in one hand, such as an arm or foot, then support it with one hand and use your other hand to make the massage movement. If, however, you are working on an area such as the back or stomach, on which you can place both hands, you can then use both hands to perform the massage.

There are two styles of movement. You may choose between them according to the contours of the area on which you are working. One movement may feel more comfortable to you than the other. Or you may combine them. This is entirely a personal decision.

One style is to make movements that are smooth, even and circular. These should cover the area of the injury or pain and also circle around the entire surrounding skin area. You can move your hand in either a clockwise or counter-clockwise direction, depending on what feels most natural to you at the time.

The second style is to move your hand laterally backward and forward, just as if you were dusting a flat surface from side to side.

Use your full palm and fingers for the massage. Your touch should be pleasant and warm. The action of your hand is meant to be soothing and reassuring.

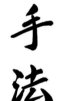

Dispersing Bruises

If you receive a heavy blow or injury on your body, a bruise normally forms. The dark colour is the blood pooling in the area. In Chinese medicine this is a sign that your internal energy, which flows with your blood, is rushing to the injured spot to protect you against attack. It is almost as if the injury acted like a powerful magnet, attracting energy towards itself. This is one of the marvellous ways in which the body shows its natural capacity for intelligence and self-healing.

However, internal tension may cause the energy to build up to such a level that it becomes blocked in the vicinity, unable to move. It is like a traffic jam. The evidence is the stagnant blood, the swelling and the pain.

You can use your energy, with Earth and Wood energy massage techniques, to release the tension in the area and disperse the blocked, excess energy.

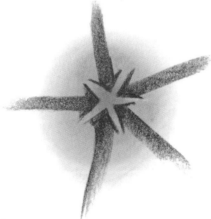

1. Metal energy
The movement of your internal energy toward the bruised area corresponds exactly to the motion described as "Metal". Energy flows from the surrounding tissues to the place where it is needed. This is the inward movement of Metal energy, like a caravan closing in on itself for protection against hostile outer forces.

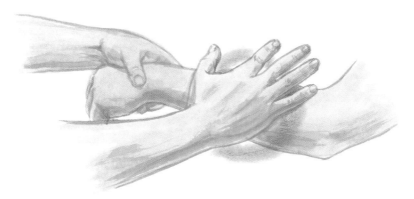

2. Earth energy

*Chi Kung massage always begins with raising your own energy
level, as described on pages 112–13. Then, support the
injured area with one hand, if this is possible, or place your
supporting hand on the opposite side of the body to the bruise.
The first strokes should be the calming, slow circular
movements of Earth energy. Keep your hands open and
relaxed. Make a dozen slow circles.*

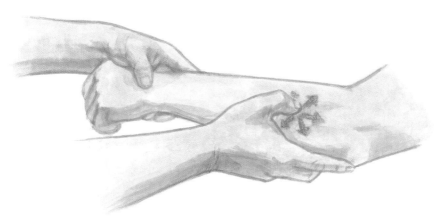

3. Wood energy

*The purpose of the massage is to disperse any energy that is
not needed for healing purposes and which may be causing
congestion in the area under the skin. You influence this
blockage by moving your own energy in a pattern which moves
outward from the centre. This is the pattern of Wood energy.
Place your hand so that your thumb can work steadily and
firmly around the area, drawing the energy outward.*

Tending Twists and Sprains

We feel the pain of a twisted or sprained joint when a sharp, sudden movement pulls and tears muscle, tendon or ligament fibres. The internal injury often produces internal bleeding in the area, accompanied by visible and very tender swelling.

When this happens, Chi spontaneously flows toward the injured joint. As the additional energy builds up, it generates heat. A sort of air lock forms around the area, creating a tiny oven in which the heat is trapped. Food and drink that tend to constrict the flow of Chi in the joints, such as beer, hot chili, duck and vinegar, will make the condition worse.

The following massage sequence will often help to release the build-up of energy in the area, relieve the pain and reduce the swelling.

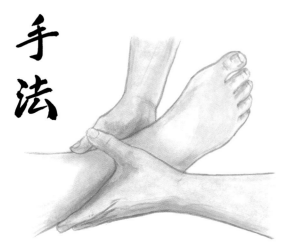

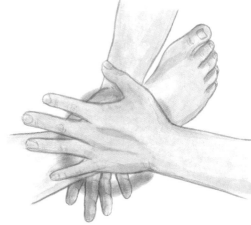

1. Two poles
After stimulating the flow of Chi to your hands (see pages 112–13), place both your hands for a minute around the affected joint. This is like enclosing the injury in a healing force field.

2. Earth energy
Support the joint with one hand. With the other hand, make smooth, calming circles around the entire area. Your touch should be warming and penetrating, but not so intense that it creates unwanted pressure or additional pain.

3. Water energy

In order to reduce the swelling in the area, place your hand directly over the injury and make sustained vibrations downward, as if sending signals inward from the skin to the muscle and bone.

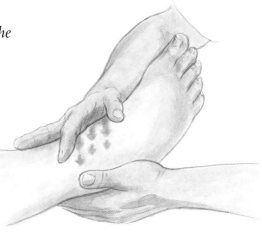

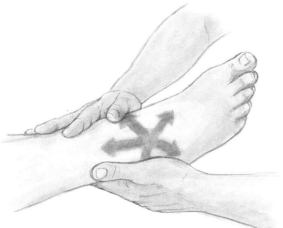

4. Wood energy

To disperse excess energy that has accumulated and become blocked around the joint, use your palm to make a series of firm strokes that radiate outward from the area. If the injury is not too tender, you may be able to make these movements with your thumb.

5. Earth energy

Finally, complete the massage with smooth and soothing circular movements, with both hands over the entire area.

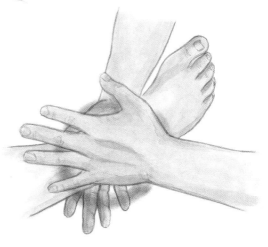

Alleviating Backaches

Among the most common causes of backache are muscle strains resulting from heavy lifting, injuries caused by falls or other accidents, and inappropriate movements affecting the alignment of the spine. Backache can result from prolonged poor posture and may also reflect mental and emotional disturbances and other types of stress.

If there has been a structural problem in the spine, such as a slipped disc, specialist treatment is needed. A Chi Kung expert, using the following sequence, will perform certain corrective manipulations of the spine in between the different types of massage. However, if you or a family member is suffering from less aggravated stiffness and pain in the back, you may be able to help each other with this sequence on its own.

1. Two poles
After stimulating the flow of Chi to your hands (see pages 112–13), rest both your hands for a minute on either side of the area of the back where the pain is located.

2. Earth energy
Start to move both your hands in calm circles over the whole area surrounding the pain. This reduces tension in the flesh and muscles and helps calm the person's mind. Without this relaxation, it will be harder to work on the muscles in the area.

3. Wood and water energy

Resting one hand comfortably on the person's back for support, use your other hand to make firm, vibrating movements that radiate outward from the area of pain. The vibration should be done as if the successive pressures were sinking into the back (Water movement) and the movements should aim to draw excess energy away from the area (Wood movement).

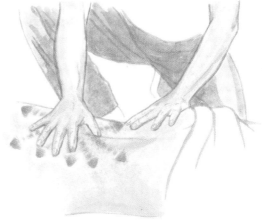

4. Fire energy

The back is so strong that the site of the energy blockage and pain is normally very deep. Press your whole hand directly over the pain and then withdraw it suddenly, like a plunger unblocking a drain. Do this several times.

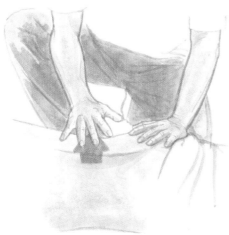

5. Earth energy

Complete the massage with smooth and soothing circular movements, with both hands over the entire area.

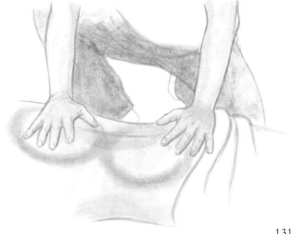

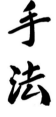

Relieving Headaches

There are many causes for headaches, but the result is either that there is a tremendous upward rush of energy into the head or that there is a blockage of the energy flow to and from the head. Some pains in the head are the result of accidents and injuries – these require specialist treatment. But most ordinary headaches are caused by a blockage or stagnation of Chi in the area of the neck and shoulders, which affects the supply of blood and oxygen to the brain. You can use the following sequence yourself to help relieve your own headaches, or you can try using it to help your friends or family.

1. Earth and Water energy
Begin by massaging the temples. Work with the tips of two or three fingers on each temple. Make smooth circles around the area of the temples (Earth energy), pressing gently inward (Water energy). Complete 36 small circles.

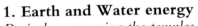

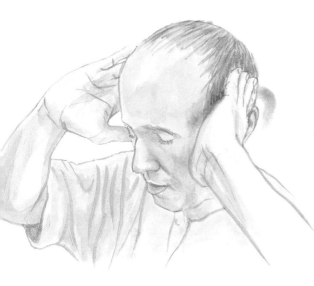

2. Wood energy
To release the blockage of Chi, firmly run your fingers along both sides of the head from the temples, behind the ears and down to the base of the skull at the neck. Let your fingertips press firmly into the bony structure of the skull as they trace the path from the temples to the neck. Repeat this flowing motion half a dozen times.

3. Earth and Water energy
Massage both sides of the neck. Work with the tips of two or three fingers on either side of the back of the neck, below the base of the skull. Make 36 small circles (Earth energy), pressing gently inward as you move (Water energy).

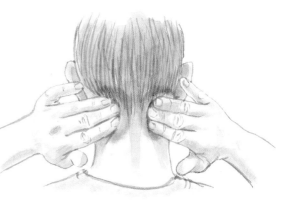

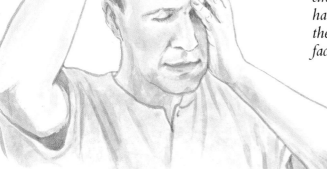

4. Earth energy
Rub your hands together until they are warm. Then "wash" your head and face with your hands. Use firm and smooth circular movements, with your hands moving continuously over the entire surface of your head and face for about a minute.

反樸歸真

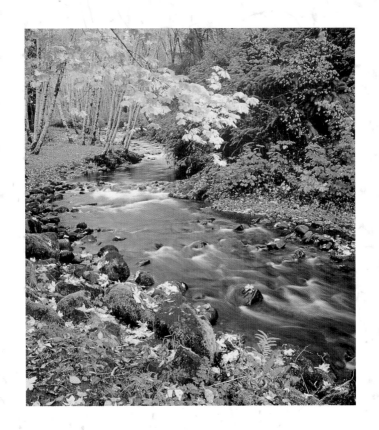

PART FIVE

RETURNING
TO THE
SOURCE

Recovering your Health

Introduction

*The restoration of energy is all a matter of stabilizing
nature. If you can be stable in nature, then energy will
spontaneously return. It cannot be forced.*

LIU I-MING

When you feel ill or weak, it is often because you have
low levels of energy in your system. You may feel phys-
ically drained, and you may also find yourself feeling
listless, depressed or confused. All these unpleasant
effects can be the result of having a depleted energy
reservoir. In other words, the vital energy in your Tan
Tien (see pages 26–7) is too low.

This energy depletion corresponds to the symbolic
representations described on pages 11–12:

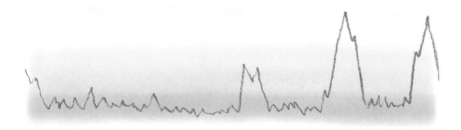

There can be many reasons for this condition. Your
energy may have been completely run down as a result
of physical and mental stress. It may have been used up
fighting an infection. You could be emotionally
fatigued.

Sometimes, there can be a blockage in the circulation of
energy somewhere in your body, so there is an excess of
energy in one part of your system and far too little left
elsewhere in your body. A common example is the
migraine headache: there is pounding, intense energy

blocked in the head, while the rest of the body is left weak and exhausted.

Ordinary exercise is the very last thing you feel able to do. You don't even have the energy to go for a walk. This is when the internal energy work of Chi Kung can be extremely helpful.

In this part of the book you are shown how to do the fundamental practices that will help replenish your lost reserves of Chi and how to stimulate the flow of that energy through your body. These can be done while lying in bed, sitting or using various forms of physical support.

On the path to recovery, you will likely find that there are times when you feel ready to start doing the basic exercises in the standing positions shown in Part One. Be careful not to rush ahead, as even this form of practice can tire you out if you are not ready for it.

If you need support while standing up, try leaning your back against a wall. But if you find that it takes too much effort to get to your feet, or you feel dizzy or unstable while standing, then you can return to using a sitting position or, if necessary, practising while lying down as shown in the following pages.

From time to time you may feel too weak to be able to continue with the standing exercises at all. This sense of tiredness need not be merely the result of physical weariness. You might be feeling some sense of emotional depletion. Simply return to doing the same practices, either using a wall for support, or sitting or lying down.

Try not to abandon your Chi Kung training. It is meant to accompany you on your journey, both when you are feeling positive within yourself and when you are facing great difficulties.

The Immortals

These three figures, known as The Immortals, express our desire for health, happiness and good fortune. Whether we are well or ill, these desires seem to be perpetual. They shape generation after generation. As individuals we are mortal, but our aspirations transcend our lifespan.

The figure on the left symbolizes Happiness. He is shown holding a child, the fruition of sexual union and the future hope of the family.

The central figure is dressed in the robes of a high official in the imperial court. He holds a sceptre, without which he would not be admitted into the presence of the emperor. This figure represents Good Fortune – success and prosperity in all undertakings.

The figure on the right embodies the idea of Long Life. He holds a freshly cut branch of ripe peaches, an ancient symbol of longevity. The aspiration is not merely to die at an old age, but to live a life of continuous health and well-being, always filled with the life force.

The imposing wooden sculpture of The Immortals on the facing page was hand carved in China and may date back centuries. The quality of the work suggests that it may have been the lifetime's achievement of a single sculptor. It was hidden in a small kitchen to prevent its destruction during the infamous Cultural Revolution. It now graces The Immortals restaurant in London's Chinatown.

Our profound desire for Happiness, Good Fortune and a Long Life manifests the life force within us. It is the signature of our Chi. When we practise Chi Kung, that force is strengthened, lifting our spirits and regenerating our inner vitality.

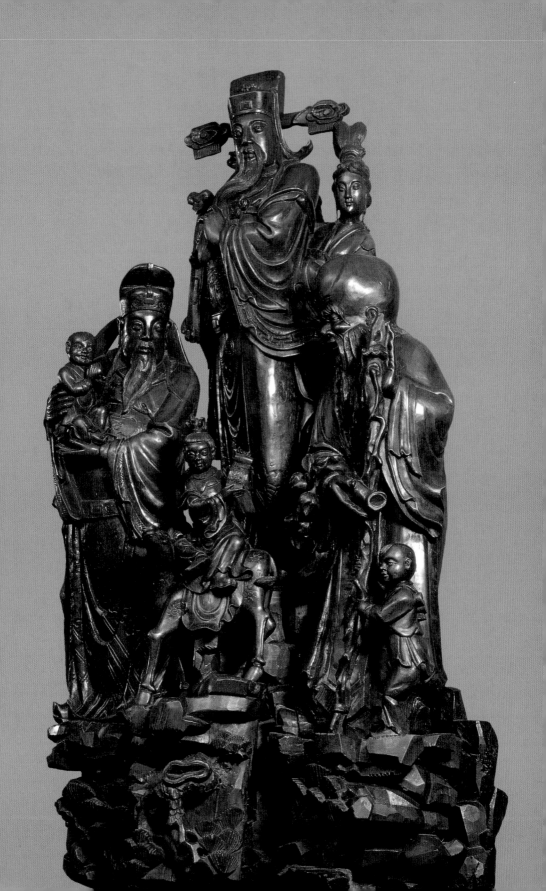

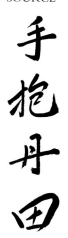

Gathering your Chi

You may be someone who is in bed because you are temporarily ill. You may be recuperating from an illness or an operation. Or you may have a condition that leaves you frequently weak and exhausted. Whatever the reason, if you are bedbound there is still a way in which you can use this time to restore your Chi.

The way you think about your condition exercises a powerful effect on your well-being. It is helpful to see yourself as undergoing a period of invisible regeneration. Like someone in retreat, you are cut off from your normal activities. It is as if you had returned to the womb: you are dwelling in a space where inner growth takes place.

If you are weak, your energy may be thinly dispersed throughout your body. In this case, the most important thing is to conserve and centre whatever energy resources you have. The way to do this is to place your hands in the position for Gathering your Chi (see pages 26–7).

Try to place your right hand over your lower abdomen. If you rest the side of your thumb lightly on your navel, your palm will fall naturally into place. Then rest your left hand comfortably on top of your right hand.

If you cannot place your hands on top of your belly, you can rest them so that they touch the sides of your abdomen. Do this as often as you can, whether awake or asleep. But do not strain yourself. Just adopt this position in a relaxed manner whenever possible.

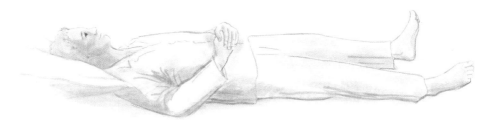

If you are feeling too weak to get out of bed, or you have been ordered to remain in bed, you can use the time to practise Gathering your Chi. If possible, lie with your back flat on the bed, placing your hands over your lower abdomen. You can do this as long as you feel able to while sleeping or dozing, or while you are awake.

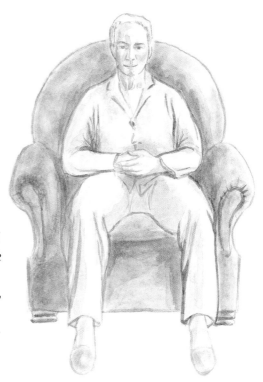

When you have regained a little strength and feel able to get out of bed, trying sitting in a comfortable chair to do this exercise. Try to avoid a chair or sofa which causes your back to slump too much, as that will compress your internal organs. Relax, place your hands over your abdomen and let your energy slowly regenerate.

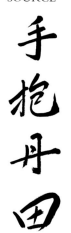

Strengthening your Chi

Even if you are still spending a great deal of time in bed, you can work with the following sequence of Chi Kung positions which will help you progressively strengthen your Chi.

There are five positions. The slight variations between each represent increasing levels of development. Since everyone's capacity varies, it is best for each individual to work with this sequence in a very personal way. If you are ill or feeling weak, your capacity will vary at different times. Sometimes you will be able to make a lot of progress and at other times you will feel you are possibly slipping backward. This is completely normal. Simply adjust the way you use these positions, according to your own feelings at the time.

You can use these positions flexibly. You can begin with the first position. If you feel comfortable holding it for up to five minutes and want to continue, move on to the second position and try to sustain it for a further five minutes. If you then progress on to the third position, but find it too strenuous, you can simply go back to the second or first position and continue for a few minutes before you end. You can apply this flexibility across the full range of five positions. There is no need to force yourself beyond your natural comfort in any position.

While in the positions, devote yourself to the healing power of relaxation. Begin with your eyes, jaws and neck. Then proceed with your shoulders and arms, feeling that they are sinking toward the floor – but not losing their position. Relax your chest and feel your entire lower body sinking into the bed. Imagine that warm light streams from your head and upper body down to the soles of your feet.

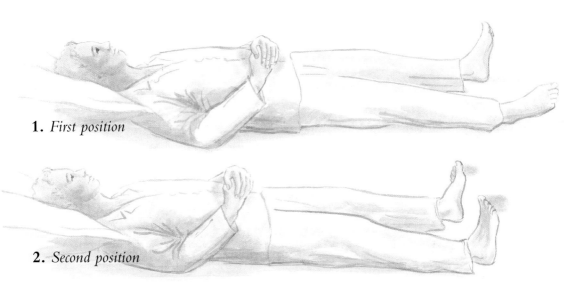

1. *First position*

2. *Second position*

1. First position. *Place both hands over your belly (see previous pages) or rest them so that they are able to rest against your abdomen. This position conserves and centres your vital energy.*

2. Second position. *Hands still on your belly. Pull your toes up, keeping your heels on the bed. This stimulates the flow of energy in your body. When your leg muscles tire, rest. Repeat when you feel able.*

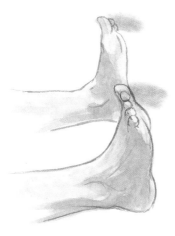

The second position (above) and the fifth position (page 145) involve pulling your toes up so that your heels rest on the bed and your toes point upward. This position works your lower leg muscles. Keep your feet in this position as long as you can – maybe only a few seconds at first, if you are very weak. Then relax your feet. Repeat as often as you wish, trying to sustain the position a little longer each time.

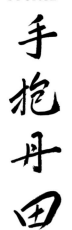

Strengthening your Chi: *next levels*

Once you are able to sustain the second position (page 143), with your toes pulled up for a few minutes, and you feel able to proceed to the next levels, you can try working with the sequence on the facing page, adjusting it to your own capacity. If you feel comfortable with one level, try increasing to the next, going up and down the levels according to your changing condition.

Your capacity will probably change from day to day. Sometimes you will only be able to hold a position for a short time. Never force yourself to stay in any position longer than feels appropriate. Remember that the effort required on any particular day may be exactly what is needed to further unblock your Chi.

3. Third position. *Hands remain on your belly. Bend your knees by drawing your feet up toward you so that your soles remain flat on the bed. This increases the flow of energy. When tired, relax completely back into a flat resting position.*

4. Fourth position. *Bend your knees as in the third position. Hold a balloon slightly above your belly, fingers apart. Rest your elbows on the bed. This strengthens and calms your energy. When tired, lower hands over your belly and relax.*

5. Fifth position. *Knees bent. Pull your toes up. Hold the balloon slightly above your belly. Lift your elbows off the bed. This raises your energy to a new level. When tired, slowly lower elbows and toes. Then rest hands over your belly and relax.*

At the conclusion of any of the positions in this sequence, you can calmly return to the position Gathering your Chi, with your right hand over your lower abdomen and your left hand on top. If you cannot maintain that position for any reason, lie comfortably with your hands resting against your abdomen.

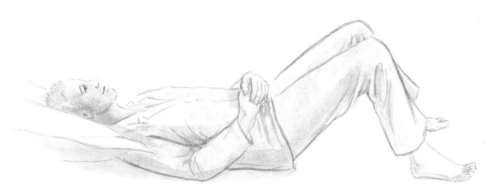

3. *Third position.*

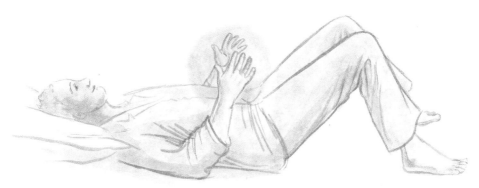

4. *Fourth position.*

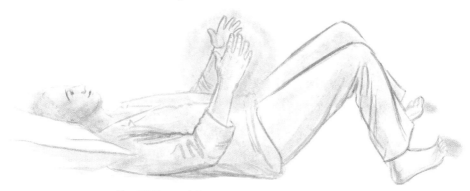

5. *Fifth position.*

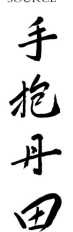

Filling your Reservoir

If you feel ready to try something a bit stronger than holding your hands over your abdomen, you can experiment with holding an imaginary Golden Sphere in front of your belly while sitting up in bed or sitting in a chair.

If you are in bed, raise yourself up so that you are sitting in a position with a fairly straight back. You can use firm cushions to give you maximum support. You do not need to be sitting upright, but try to lie so that your back is reasonably straight rather than curved.

If you are able to use a chair, choose one in which your back is fairly straight. Try not to sink down, which causes your back to become hunched and your chest to compress inward. As your energy recovers, you will find that you have the strength to sit up straighter.

Place your hands as if they were holding a large Golden Sphere in your lap. Be sure to keep your fingers slightly apart, but not tense. You can rest the backs of your hands on your thighs, or, if you feel strong enough, you can try raising your hands a little bit above your thighs.

Simply rest in that position as long as you feel able to. You can do this either in a quiet environment or to soft music. Having an open window in the room will help, as long as it is does not make the room too cold and drafty.

At other times, you can watch television, listen to the radio or talk to friends and family while sitting in a relaxed manner holding the sphere.

*As you sit calmly holding
an imaginary Golden
Sphere, your hands act like
magnets, silently attracting
healing energy toward you
from your entire
environment.*

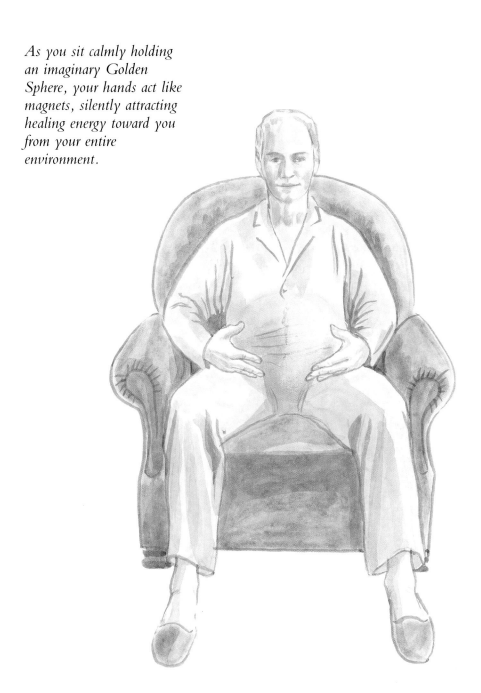

Drawing Silk from the Cocoon

Once you have practised Gathering your Chi (pages 140–1) and Strengthening your Chi (pages 142–5), you can try this next exercise to help increase the flow of Chi through your body. It is based on the version shown on pages 52–3, but is adapted for people who have difficulty standing.

You may have a condition or injury that seriously restricts the movement of your lower limbs, or be so weakened after an illness that you cannot stand up. Then, either sit in a chair or raise yourself up in bed, trying to keep your spine reasonably straight. If necessary, put a small pillow behind your lower back to support your lower spine. Perform the movement, following the same instructions, imagining that you are standing.

As you perform this movement, your internal energy will naturally begin to flow outward from its reservoir in your abdomen until it extends throughout your body – down to your feet and out to your fingertips. Let your body remain relaxed, move slowly and continuously. Rest your mind on the sensation of drawing the silk filaments calmly and carefully from the cocoon.

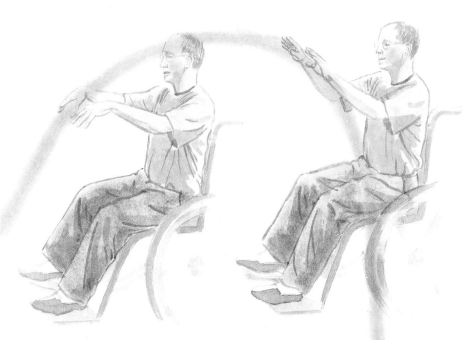

This exercise takes its name from the ancient practice of extracting raw silk from the cocoon. Imagine that a delicate thread is attached to each of your fingertips and you are going to unreel it from the cocoon without a break. It requires care, attention and steady pressure.

Begin by placing both hands slightly in front of your belly, with palms downward. If you are sitting, your palms will be a few inches above your thighs. Imagine you are reeling silk with your fingertips. As you breathe in, make a long, slow, upward stroke. Relax the shoulders and arms. The upward stroke finishes when your hands are level with your head, fingertips angled upward. As you breathe out, make a long downward stroke, until your hands are at waist level. Then make this movement continuous until you can perform it without tension for several minutes at a time.

First Movements

It takes time to restore your energy to the point where
it is full, stable and resilient. If the restoration is not
done properly you may find your internal batteries
running down over and over again. It is better to make
a little regenerative progress each day by doing the
stationary Chi Kung practices while sitting or lying
down (see pages 140–8) and, when you begin to feel
able, practising Drawing Silk from the Cocoon (see
pages 148–9). When you have recovered the strength to
do these without feeling any strain or difficulty, then
start practising the next three movement exercises.

Begin by following the instructions which show you
how the movements can be adapted for your needs.
You may also find it helpful to refer back to the
instructions given for each exercise in Part One of this
book to see if there are any aspects of the original
postures or movements that you can try as your energy
becomes stronger.

If you are ill or convalescing and are working with this
book without the benefit of a qualified teacher, you
need to pay careful attention to the subtle messages your
body sends you when you start these exercises. The
most common problem that many people experience is
impatience: you so desperately want to be fit and well
that you push yourself harder and faster than is wise.
The short-term results can be encouraging – a burst of
energy for a few hours or days. But the effect does not
last long and your energy can quickly drain away.

When you feel the time is right, and depending on your
own personal circumstances, you can decide to attempt
the exercises in the free-standing positions shown in
Part One. But if, at any point, you feel that this is too
stressful for you, simply return to the adapted form of
the exercises given here and allow your body more time
to complete its internal work.

Arousing your Chi

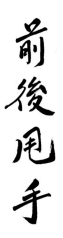

Gently swinging your arms back and forth is a
fundamental exercise for health because it stimulates the
flow of Chi along all the energy pathways of the body.
It is used in Chi Kung hospitals in China for the
treatment of many serious disorders and for convalescing
patients. It is usually done in a standing position,
without support (see pages 28–9), but it can also be
done while sitting or resting against a back support.

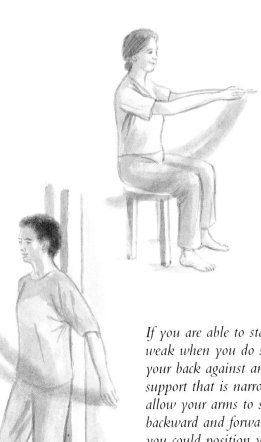

*Swing both your arms loosely
forward. Your fingers are gently
spread. Let them swing back slightly
away from your body until they
naturally stop. Let the momentum of
the swing carry them forward again.
Build up a spontaneous, gentle
swinging motion, like a rapidly
moving pendulum. If your arms are
weak or painful, don't strain them.
Even slight back and forth movements
will help. Do as many as you feel
able to, working up to 50. When
you are stronger, progress gradually
up to 200.*

*If you are able to stand but feel
weak when you do so, try resting
your back against any form of stable
support that is narrow enough to
allow your arms to swing freely
backward and forward. For example,
you could position yourself against
the inner edge of a door frame so
that your arms swing on either side
without obstruction.*

Increasing your inner warmth

When we are cold, we often slap ourselves to get warm. Coldness in Chinese medicine can be a sign that our Chi is weak, sluggish or blocked. We use this exercise to get our Chi moving more strongly. It can be done in a standing position (see pages 30–1), but will also be effective if done with the back resting against a wall, while sitting or lying.

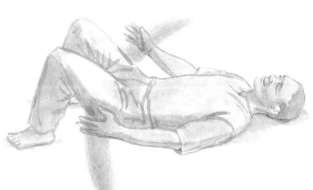

Sit on a stool or chair without arms. Relax your upper body. Make sure that your shoulders are free from tension so that your arms can hang loosely by your sides. Look straight forward with a calm gaze. Then begin slapping the outside of your thighs with the relaxed palms of your hands. The slapping should be done with a friendly feeling toward yourself and not so hard that you hurt yourself. Breathe naturally. Stop when you wish, slowly working up to 30 slaps.

You can do this exercise in bed, either lying flat or with your knees raised. In either position, you will normally still be able to slap the outside of your thighs.

Raising your internal power

This exercise (see pages 32–3) uses pressure on the sole of your foot to pump Chi through your body. You can adapt this movement to meet your present state of health, while sitting or using a table or chair for support.

Stand beside a table or place a chair beside you. Rest your hand on the table or the back of the chair and use it for support while you do the exercise.

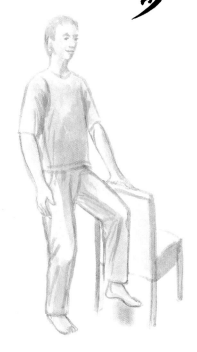

Stand with your feet facing forward, shoulder-width apart. Shift your weight on to your right foot. Imagine all your weight sinking down through the right side of your body into the ground. Then lift your left foot, trying to keep the sole parallel to the floor. Raise it only as far as you can manage without strain. As you lift your leg, breathe in. Then, as you breathe out, gently lower your left foot back down to the ground. Now shift your weight over to your left foot. Gently lift and lower your right leg in the same way. Begin with 6 alternate liftings and lowerings and build up to 12. Then stand still, with your weight evenly spread over both feet, for one minute.

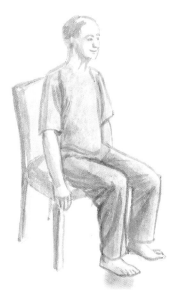

You can adapt this exercise for sitting on the edge of a chair. Sit as far forward as possible. Look forward. Press one foot down into the floor and lift the other one slightly off the ground. Breathe in as you raise the foot, breathe out as you lower it. Then slowly repeat, alternating between the feet, trying to do 6 of each and building gradually up to 12.

153

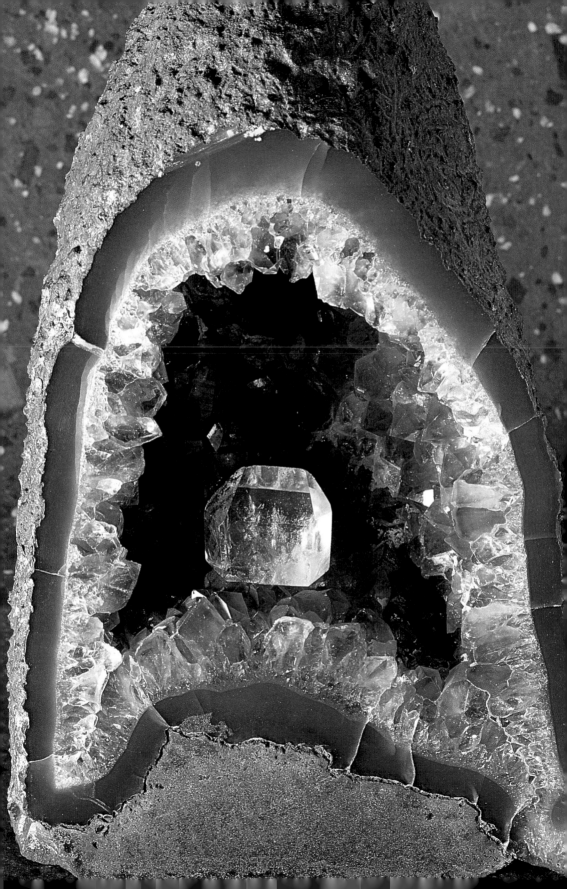

Crystal

Healing properties have long been attributed to crystals. In ancient China, people with serious illnesses received treatments which included lying on a bed of crystal. The extraordinarily strong vibrations emanating from the structure were understood to have great therapeutic value.

Most people can feel the vibration of a crystal simply by holding one in their hands. As an energy source, some types of crystal are so reliable that they are now used in timepieces and rocket guidance systems.

The special properties of natural crystals derive from the way they have formed and lain in the earth over the ages. They vibrate with the life-sustaining energy of the earth itself. Some emit positive energy, which stimulates feelings of well-being in a person. Other crystals act as transformers, absorbing harmful vibrations from the environment and converting them to positive energy patterns.

One way of increasing the power of a crystal is to place it inside an open section of rock crystal, as shown on the page opposite. Motionless, the smaller crystal begins to interact with the surrounding crystalline structures and draws power from them.

You can think of the healing processes described in this book in the same way. The Sea of Energy in your Tan Tien is like the small, clear crystal placed inside the mother crystal of your body. From the first moment of life, it is imbued with a natural healing power of its own. Through the sustained practice of Chi Kung, that power increases. Over time, the entire substance of your body is purified and your being, like a living crystal, becomes a radiant field of energy.

The Zhan Zhuang tradition and Master Lam

The Zhan Zhuang Chi Kung lineage has a history stretching back more than 2,000 years. It was not until this century that it was taught in public. Previously the art was transmitted only in secret. The Great Grand Master who brought it into the open was Wang Xiang Zhai (pronounced Wang Shang Jai) who, from his earliest youth, travelled for years throughout China learning from the great masters of his day.

The current Grand Master is Professor Yu Yong Nian in Beijing who studied directly under Great Grand Master Wang. Professor Yu is the world's leading authority on the system and has written four books on the subject. The first sold 100,000 copies in China and the others are now collectors' items. As a result of his work and under his direction, the health-giving properties of Zhan Zhuang have been formally acknowledged by hospitals throughout China and introduced into patient care.

Professor Yu is an honorary member of the Council of the Association of Chi Kung Science of the People's Republic of China and adviser to the American-Chinese Chi Kung Association.

上述源流简介完全正确。林锦全是我的亲传弟子。是他首先将东方古来的健身之法、站桩疗法介绍到西方世界。一九九〇年我去伦敦时亲眼见到了一些经过现代西方医学久治不愈的病人，林锦全用东方中国的站桩疗法治愈了他们的顽疾。他们对林锦全和我表示了尊敬和感激之意。林锦全向西方世界传播东方文化，对东西方医学交流，取长补短，造福人类，作出先一贡献。

In the handwritten statement reproduced here, Professor Yu writes: "Lam Kam Chuen is my disciple. It is he who first took the Asian-Chinese health system, Zhan Zhuang, to the West. In 1990 I visited London where I saw for myself people who had been treated with Western medicine without success; Lam Kam Chuen used our Zhan Zhuang therapy to help restore their health. These people were very grateful not only towards him, but to me as well, and presented their respect and thanks. Lam Kam Chuen came to the West, presented our system and introduced this art in a way that created an interchange between Eastern and Western health and medical systems."

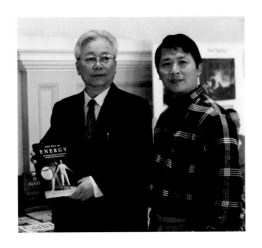

The Zhan Zhuan tradition is now being established beyond the Chinese-speaking world. In 1991 Gaia Books published Master Lam's ground-breaking work, *The Way of Energy*. Professor Yu, seen here with Master Lam at a pre-publication event in Gloucestershire, has followed its progress closely. The work is now available in many languages worldwide.

Master Lam writes: "At an early age in Hong Kong I was introduced to classical Chinese arts. Day by day, as I trained in Zhan Zhuang, I could feel its benefits. Eventually it was my good fortune to be able to study in Beijing directly under Professor Yu Yong Nian. Professor Yu shared his immense experience with me, freely opening up his understanding and the results of his experiments in combining Chi Kung with Western medicine. From the research we conducted together, he made it possible for me to derive the full benefits of Zhan Zhuang in my life and to explore its depths. I am convinced that this art can help people regardless of boundaries and I have devoted myself to opening up its wonders to the world."

我年青時在香港,對中國古文化很有興趣,學習研究,接觸到"站樁"功法,練後感覺舒適又甜美,身體更強健。故專誠到北京拜在于永年老師門下深造。多年來得于老師言傳身教無私地將他畢生研習所得,有系統地傳授給我合我獲益良多。幾年前,我業餘用站樁功法,在歐洲推廣,教人用以治病、防病,收效良好。故希為人類健康盡一份力量。往後日子裏,將站樁功推向全世界。

Anyone wishing to contact Master Lam for advice, instruction or workshops is welcome to do so. Please write to Master Lam Kam Chuen, The Immortals, Second Floor, 58–60 Shaftesbury Avenue, London W1V 7DE. Mobile phone: (44) 0831 802 598. Fax: (44) (171) 437 3118.

INDEX

Acknowledgements

Author's acknowledgements

I would like to thank my wife, Kai Sin, who has supported me over the years and made it possible to concentrate on developing my practice and teaching of Zhan Zhuang and Chinese medicine. I am also grateful to my three boys, Tin Yun, Tin Yu and Tin Hun. Tin Hun especially has persevered along with me in experimenting with Chi Kung and has helped me greatly in my understanding.

The leaders of Gaia Books, Joss Pearson, Pip Morgan and Patrick Nugent, have been present and helpful throughout the birth of this book and given me the freedom to present these teachings exactly as I wished.

I would like to apologise to Bridget Morley, the designer, for the very difficult demands we have placed upon her and to express my delight at the final result.

A special word of appreciation goes to my students who have persisted in the study of Zhan Zhuang and Tai Chi with patience and devotion and become the foundation on which future teaching in the West will be based.

Finally, I would like to thank my student, Richard Reoch. Working with him has enabled me to communicate the essence of these arts to a much wider audience than might otherwise have been possible. Together we have tried to build bridges between the cultures of East and West and between the rich legacy of the past and the unfolding potential of the present.

Publisher's acknowledgements

Gaia Books would like to thank Master Lam and his wife Kai Sin for their unlimited hospitality and patience during the production of this book. They would also like to thank Sara Mathews for her helpful suggestions, Angela Casey of Broadway Books for her insightful comments on the draft text and Bryony Allen for the index.

Photo credits

Deni Bown, all pictures of Master Lam Kam Chuen performing Chi Kung; Ardea London Ltd, p. 21, Ron and Valerie Taylor; Bridgeman Art Library, pp. 114, 120, Shield, ordered by Green, War & Green for presentation by the Merchants and Bankers of the City to the Duke of Wellington, designed by Thomas Stothard, made by Benjamin Smith, c.1822 (silver); Aspley House, The Wellington Museum, London/Bridgeman Art Library, London/New York; Oxford Scientific Films, p. 104, Isaac Kehimkar Dinodia; Science Photo Library, p. 8, Julian Baum, p. 84, Erich Schrempp, p. 107, NASA, pp. 114, 118, Sinclair Stammers; Stock Market Photo Agency Inc., pp. 47, 75, 135; Tony Stone Images Ltd, pp. 115, 122, Richard Elliott, pp. 115, 120, Rich Iwasaki; Sam Scott-Hunter, pp. 124, 138, 154.